Total
Reflexology
of the
Hand

"*Total Reflexology of the Hand* is a 'must-have' for all reflexologists seeking to deepen their knowledge and take their practice to whole new levels. It is elegant and insightful in its holistic approach to integrating the brain-body with the cranial concept in hand reflexology. This book is a joy to read and learn from. I highly recommend it."

CAROL FAGUY, RCRT/MCSRI, TEACHER WITH CRANIO-SACRAL
REFLEXOLOGY INTERNATIONAL ACADEMY OF EXCELLENCE
AND REFLEXOLOGY ASSOCIATION OF CANADA

"This is a complementary approach that we can use in our practice to help our patients. Thanks to Martine for always giving us a bigger picture of our practice and more tools to handle it as professionals and caregivers."

EMMANUELLE RUEN-HAYES, CERTIFIED REFLEXOLOGIST

Total
Reflexology
of the
Hand

An Advanced Guide to the Integration of Craniosacral Therapy and Reflexology

Martine Faure-Alderson, D.O.

Translated by Jon E. Graham

Healing Arts Press
Rochester, Vermont • Toronto, Canada

Healing Arts Press
One Park Street
Rochester, Vermont 05767
www.HealingArtsPress.com

Healing Arts Press is a division of Inner Traditions International

Originally published in French under the title *Réflexologie thérapie totale de la main: Du réflexe à la conscience* by Guy Trédaniel Éditeur
First U.S. edition published in 2016 by Healing Arts Press

Note to the reader: *This book is intended as an informational guide. The remedies, approaches, and techniques described herein are meant to supplement, and not to be a substitute for, professional medical care or treatment. They should not be used to treat a serious ailment without prior consultation with a qualified health care professional.*

Library of Congress Cataloging-in-Publication Data
Names: Faure-Alderson, Martine.
Title: Total reflexology of the hand : an advanced guide to the integration of craniosacral therapy and reflexology / Martine Faure-Alderson, D.O. ; translated by Jon E. Graham.
Other titles: Râeflexologie thâerapie totale de la main. English
Description: First U.S. edition. | Rochester, Vermont : Healing Arts Press, [2016] | Translation of
French title: Râeflexologie thâerapie totale de la main : du râeflexe áa la conscience, 2014. | Includes bibliographical references and index.
Identifiers: LCCN 2015046800 (print) | LCCN 2015050111 (e-book) | ISBN 9781620555316 (pbk.) | ISBN 9781620555323 (e-book)
Subjects: LCSH: Reflexology (Therapy) | Hand--Massage. | Hand exercises.
Classification: LCC RM723.R43 F3713 2016 (print) | LCC RM723.R43 (e-book) | DDC 615.8/224—dc23
LC record available at http://lccn.loc.gov/2015046800

Printed and bound in India by Replika Press Pvt. Ltd.

10 9 8 7 6 5 4 3 2 1

Text design and layout by Virginia Scott Bowman
This book was typeset in Garamond Premier Pro with Perpetua, Helvetica, and Avenir used as display typefaces

To send correspondence to the author of this book, mail a first-class letter to the author c/o Inner Traditions • Bear & Company, One Park Street, Rochester, VT 05767, and we will forward the communication, or visit **www.craniosacralreflexologyinternational.com**.

Contents

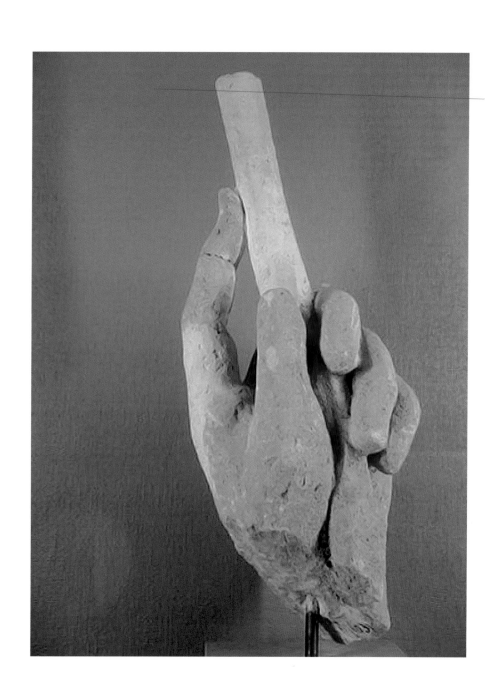

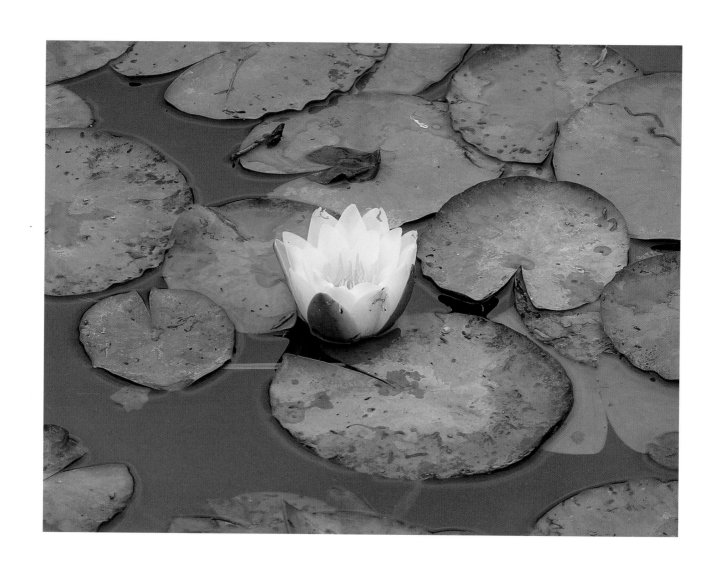

PART ONE

Introduction to Reflexology

It is because he has hands that man is most intelligent.

ANAXAGORAS

History

The healing art of reflexology is thousands of years old. The Chinese employed acupressure therapy some five thousand years ago, and by approximately 2,500 BCE they had divided the body into longitudinal meridians, as found in the traditional Chinese medicine practice of acupuncture. Likewise, the ancient Egyptians were familiar with a form of therapeutic massage of the feet and hands, as shown in a fresco found on a Sixth Dynasty tomb in Saqqarah that depicts two men receiving this kind of treatment on their hands and feet.

Moving forward, in 1582 two European physicians, a Dr. Adamus and Dr. A'tatis, together published a book devoted to zone therapy. A year later, in 1583, in Leipzig, a Dr. Bell wrote a book on the technique of "pressure therapy" that was practiced at that time in Central Europe among all classes, from peasants to courtiers. A form of reflexology also existed among tribal peoples of Africa, America, and Australia.

In the nineteenth century there was a flurry of scientific interest in the field that came to be known as reflexology. In 1886, the noted neurologists Henry Head, John Hughlings Jackson, and Charles Sherrington founded the Neurological Society of London, one of seventeen societies that merged with the Medical and Chirurgical Society of London to form the current Royal Society of Medicine, to encourage the collection and exchange of ideas on all matters concerning the human brain and nervous system. In 1893, Head further developed one of Jackson's ideas, which viewed the nervous system as consisting of layers, in which each layer is covered by a higher layer. While treating patients suffering from spinal cord lesions, Head discovered sensitized zones on the skin surface that were connected to certain illnesses of the internal organs. He used his discoveries to draw up a map now known as *Head's zones*. This map identifies the dermatomes, i.e., the areas of skin supplied with afferent nerve fibers by a single posterior spinal root. This map proves that a neurological relationship exists between the skin on the surface of the body and the body's inner organs.

Meanwhile, Head's associate Charles Sherrington (who later won the Nobel Prize in physiology in 1932) demonstrated that sensitive nerve endings collected stimulations from within the body. He coined the term *synapse* in 1897 to describe these nerve endings. These are Sherrington's fields of inter-receptor sensitivity, which became part of what has come to be known as Sherrington's law of reciprocal innervation. In 1906, Sherrington wrote *The Integrative Action of the Nervous System,* in which he explained how the brain, the spinal cord, and numerous reflex paths react and adjust to internal and external stimuli.

In Germany in the 1890s, Dr. Alfons Cornelius discovered that pressure applied to certain parts of the body, while likely following the nerve pathways, triggered mental and physical reactions such as variations in temperature and humidity, as well as alterations of blood pressure. There are more than seventeen thousand nerve endings in the feet and an equal number in the hands. It appears that by stimulating them,

The Ten Zones

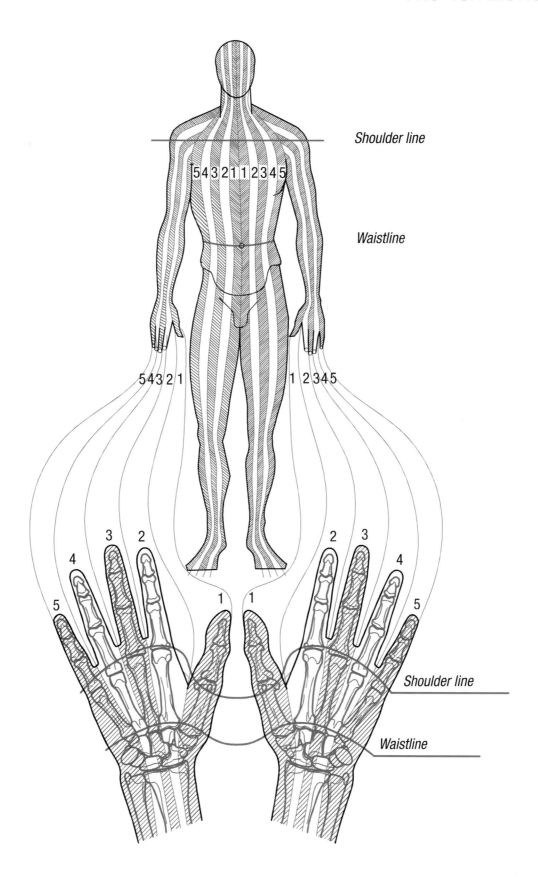

Shoulder line

Waistline

5 4 3 2 1 1 2 3 4 5

5 4 3 2 1   1 2 3 4 5

4   3   2   2   3   4

5   1   1   5

Shoulder line

Waistline

reactions are produced in the rest of the body. In 1902 he published a book titled *Pressure Points, Their Origin and Significance.*

Dr. William Fitzgerald (1872–1942), a general practitioner and ear, nose, and throat specialist who worked in Connecticut after many years of working in hospitals in Paris, London, and Vienna, began studying a technique that he called *zone therapy.* Observing that some of his nose and throat operations were virtually painless for the patient, he deduced that this local anesthesia was produced by the pressure that the patient personally exerted on his or her own hand. He gradually integrated zone therapy into his practice, using it to deaden pain, thereby replacing painkillers in minor operations. In this way he treated lumps in the breast, uterine fibroids, respiratory problems, and eye conditions. Over time Fitzgerald drew up a chart in which he divided the body into ten zones (five on each side of a median dividing line), each of which terminated in a finger and a toe.

Fitzgerald's theories on reflexology would later be refined by an American physiotherapist, Eunice Ingham (1889–1974). Author of the books *Stories the Feet Can Tell, Zone Therapy and Gland Reflexes,* and *Stories the Feet Have Told,* she created plates that show the placement of the different organs on the foot. These books constitute the foundation of modern reflexology, yet are considered both too symptom-oriented and not scientific enough, as the anatomical and physiological basics are omitted.

The late Doreen Bayly was a student of Eunice Ingham. Bayly developed her own method of treatment, in which pressure is applied to reflex points with a flexed thumb or fingers using a firm but not heavy pressure. This method is less stressful on the thumb and finger joints, and the less rapid movement is considered to be more relaxing to the patient. The Bayly School of Reflexology (www.londonreflexologycentre.co.uk), the official teaching body of the British Reflexology Association, was the first reflexology school to be established in Great Britain, with Bayly herself running courses until 1966. Doreen Bayly was my teacher, and my training with her inspired the method you are about to learn in this book.

General Principles of Reflexology

Webster's Dictionary defines *reflex* as "an action or movement of the body that happens automatically as a reaction to something; something that you do without thinking as a reaction to something." This definition touches on why and how the practice of reflexology works to create healing.

The method of total reflexology therapy that I present in this book is based on the following fundamental observations:

▶ The principle of holism is the idea that systems, whether physical, biological, chemical, social, economic, mental, linguistic, etc., and their properties should be viewed as wholes, not as collections of parts. In terms of healing, this implies that everything is in everything, and that everything is the cause of everything. Holism focuses on the dynamic oneness of the body, which is intrinsically self-regulating and self-healing.

▶ The craniosacral principle, central to osteopathy, is based on the study of the fluctuations of cerebrospinal fluid that work on the nervous system by means of the primary respiratory mechanism, or PRM.

▶ When the occipital zones, whether they are structural, sympathetic, or parasympathetic, are disrupted, they are painfully sensitive to reflex mas-

sage; this is confirmation of the precise zones on the foot and hand that need to be treated.

▶ The human being is an emotional, mental, and physical (e.g., bones, muscles, nerves, organs, fluids) whole. For this reason, any treatment of a strictly physical nature applied to this or that reflex point or zone can produce an effect that goes beyond the physical and into the psychological/mental plane governing this or that area of the body, thereby triggering a healthy emotional reaction. For example, a painful reflex point that corresponds to the stomach can reveal not a food that is hard to digest, but rather a traumatizing event that is equally "indigestible," even one that occurred a long time ago.

These basic observations are rooted in rigorous scientific methodology. This means that the appropriate treatment always requires an exact diagnosis; only after the problem has been correctly diagnosed can pressure be applied to the precise corresponding points and zones of the foot and hand. This precision can only occur when one takes as references certain anatomical landmarks that are infallible and unchanging; only the human skeleton can furnish such landmarks that are necessary to achieve this precision, which can be almost microscopic. For example, this protrusion at the base of a finger, or that joining between the bones of the inside edge of the finger, hold this cardinal point or that reflex point of a specific vertebra.

Next, the reflex zones that correspond to the different regions and different systems of the human body—for example, the nervous, circulatory, or skeletomuscular systems—are mapped out and developed between these reference points. The organs and ipsilateral (on the same side) limbs whose reflex points belong to the same zone are treated simultaneously and by analogy. For example, the foot/hand, elbow/knee, and shoulder/hip are relationships that are defined as *cross-reflexes*.

Reflexology Stimulates Self-Healing

Practiced regularly, reflexology leads to a true regeneration of the body. Why? Because just like the genome, the genetic material of an organism, the human body is innately capable of self-healing because it possesses all the restorative and immunity factors it needs. All natural medicine therapies work on this principle, by helping the person provide a favorable environment that allows for an increase in the energy needed to restore the balance necessary for the body's systems to function harmoniously. This process is called *homeostasis*. In this way, reflexology provides an incontestable sense of well-being that helps a person withstand all the challenges of life, be they emotional, physical, or mental.

An economical therapeutic and preventive modality, reflexology makes it possible to better grasp the nature of each individual's case and understand all the disorders that may be involved. It offers an excellent adjunct to both preoperative and postoperative treatments. In chronic diseases characterized by cellular degeneration, its effect is not merely palliative but offers concrete support that compensates for the degeneration of tissues.

Indications for Use

Reflexology can have equally successful results for newborns and elderly alike—and everybody in between. There are many indications for the use of reflexology:

▶ All disorders affecting the functional, hormonal, digestive, nervous, vascular, respiratory, renal, and genital systems lend themselves to reflexology treatment.

▶ In the case of pregnancy, it is important to avoid treating certain zones, and attention must be focused on respecting the lunar calendar; otherwise reflexology can be used to soothe aches and pains in the back and can provide relief from morning sickness, heartburn, swelling in the legs (if not due to preeclampsia), constipation, high blood pressure (again, as long as it appears without the other symptoms of preeclampsia), insomnia, bladder problems, mild cramping, and even hemorrhoids.

▶ Reflexology offers invaluable assistance for tolerating both serious illnesses and the medicines required to treat them.

▶ As an adjunct therapy, reflexology is just as helpful as acupuncture, homeopathy, phytotherapy, and psychotherapy. As well, for balanced health, one should not only look to lifestyle but make sure that you get proper rest, nutrition, and physical exercise.

▶ Reflexology can be used for one who is seeking to lose weight or for the treatment of insomnia, poor digestion, painful menses, or infertility; in such cases practitioners of reflexology should always start by assessing the extent of stress the person has suffered and the degree of dysfunction or degeneration of tissues.

Advantages of Hand Reflexology

Exactly like foot reflexology, hand reflexology works on the body's energetic system by stimulating specific areas, or reflex zones, located on the hands. Each of these areas corresponds to a specific region of the body, mainly the organs and the glands. This connection with the different areas of the body is the basis of the zone concept. The stimulation of a reflex zone encourages the healing process within its corresponding region of the body by restoring the flow of energy and relieving stress, as well as by improving blood irrigation and the transmission of the synapses. Another major benefit of hand reflexology is that it establishes a deep state of relaxation conducive to healing.

Most people think of the feet when they hear the word *reflexology,* but hand reflexology offers certain distinct advantages. For example, it is quite practical when time and space factors make it impossible to work on the feet. It is also good for people who are quite ticklish, or whose feet are unduly sensitive or prone to perspiring. Furthermore, because hand reflexology is so discreet, it is possible to practice it on yourself in a public setting without attracting attention.

Distinctive Features of Total Reflexology Therapy

Reflexology acts holistically on three levels: the physical, the emotional or psychological, and the mental. We can therefore define health as:

► physical freedom, the absence of pain, a sense of well-being
► emotional freedom, serenity
► mental freedom, the relaxed exercise of all our faculties

We have inherited this notion of our triple nature from Plato, and I have retained this fundamental principle in my method of total reflexology therapy for the analytical clarity it brings to human behavior. By distinguishing these three levels—formerly identified as body, soul, and spirit—we should not forget that they are absolutely inseparable and interdependent, continuously interacting on one another. Therefore, an emotional shock such as the one caused by news of the death of a close friend or relative will first engender an unbalanced state in the person on the physical plane (tears, loss of energy, muscle fatigue, loss of appetite, digestive dysfunction). At this point a mental reaction will often intervene (reasonable analysis of the event, the desire to get past the ordeal, the decision to restore the rhythms of everyday life) that in some cases permits a return to psychic equilibrium, then finally to physical equilibrium—or the opposite.

The Emergence of Reflexology as a Viable Healing Modality

Reflexology is enjoying growing interest thanks to the broader acceptance of alternative and natural healing modalities, as well as for its effectiveness in stress management and the treatment of all kinds of diseases. There are numerous hypotheses concerning its mode of action, which involve the nervous system, pain and how it is perceived, endorphins, the energy pathways, therapeutic touch, blood circulation, the placebo effect, and, most importantly, the zone concept.

All reflexology techniques are based on the development of the sense of touch and its intelligent evaluation. This is *proprioception,* the reception of stimuli produced within the organism. This proprioceptive sense of the fingers that feel and send information to the brain on the state of the tissue involved is not something that can be acquired in a day's time. Like any healing art, much study and practical experience is necessary for a practitioner of hand reflexology to acquire this refined sense of touch, but when it is acquired it ensures that these proprioceptive feelings are intelligent and reliable. Like a finely tuned instrument, the fingers of the reflexologist will know exactly what is actually taking place, especially when the practitioner is equipped with previously visualized imagery that guides her or his feeling. In this way, the practitioner does not imagine; she or he *feels.*

For this reason, knowledge of the anatomy and physiology of the human body is necessary; it allows the reflexologist to detect, uncover, and analyze the disrupted zones, and to determine whether they are hard, tender, congested, blocked, or too relaxed—all possible symptoms that can occur when there is a hindrance in the circulation of the veins, arteries, nerves, or lymph. It is only when this analysis has been completed that the reflexologist can move from perception to applying the appropriate treatment. This is of primary importance in both craniosacral therapy and in reflexology.

The other major principle underlying hand reflexology is that of holism, the dynamic oneness of the body, which is self-regulating and self-healing. Accordingly, my method emphasizes the dominant role of the autonomic nervous system, the control system that acts largely unconsciously and regulates bodily functions such as heart rate, digestion, respiration, pupillary response, urination, and sexual arousal, as disorders in the body are often connected to autonomic nervous problems caused by stress.

Over the years, working in collaboration with my students, I have integrated the following key principles of osteopathy into my method of reflexology.

The Craniosacral System and Primary Respiratory Mechanism

The bones of the skull retract and expand, flexing and extending. The cerebrospinal fluid, which serves as a shock absorber in the brain, transmits to all the cells of the body the fluctuations that the rachis (spinal cord) nerves and autonomic nervous system transmit to the fasciae. These fluctuations of the cerebrospinal fluid work on the nervous system by means of the primary respiratory mechanism.

The PRM concept is central to osteopathy. Though primary respiration has two phases, inhalation and exhalation, this is a different concept from, and not to be confused with, secondary respiration, which refers to the more familiar process of breathing that occurs with the movement of the rib cage involving a change in volume of the lungs, with an oxygen and carbon dioxide exchange. Primary respiration is a deeper, more basic process to life. PRM can be perceived in all the body's tissues at a rate of twelve to sixteen pulsations a minute. The cerebrospinal fluid thereby strengthens the bond that exists between the body's structure, connective tissue, bones, muscles, fluids, and brain.

The Sympathetic and Parasympathetic Nervous Systems

The autonomic nervous system is made up of two antagonistic yet complementary systems, the sympathetic and the parasympathetic, which are in a constant state of self-regulation. These systems govern all internal functions that are not subject to the conscious will: respiration, digestion, elimination, and reproduction. They contribute to the body's ability to defend itself, restore, and achieve balance, thereby assuring the protection of life itself.

The sympathetic nervous system's primary process is to stimulate the body's fight-or-flight response. It is constantly active at a basic level, maintaining a state of homeostasis. The parasympathetic nervous system operates when the body is at rest, especially after eating, but also governs sexual arousal, salivation, lacrimation (tears), urination, digestion, and defecation.

Every time we feel pain, the body releases endorphins. Endorphins are neurotransmitters whose analgesic effects are comparable to the effects of morphine. The pressure applied to the zones being treated during a reflexology session also release endorphins. The signals that inform the brain about this pressure compete with those that inform it of pain. In this way, they cause a traffic jam in the lower nerve fascia of the central nervous system, creating more stimulation than the system can interpret. The result is an anesthetizing effect on the pain. It is the autonomic nervous system that transmits these reactive effects caused by reflexology, and this is why we restore homeostasis during a reflexology session.

The Stress Response

Hans Selye (1907–1982) was an endocrinologist who conducted pioneering work on what has become known as the *stress response,* the nonspecific response of an organism to stressors. He posited that stress is a major cause of disease because chronic stress causes long-term chemical changes to the body. In his general adaptation syndrome model, he described three phases of the effects of stress on the body:

In the first stage, the alarm stage, your initial reaction to stress is to recognize there is a danger and you prepare to deal with the threat, i.e., the fight-or-flight response. In the second phase, the resistance stage, the source of stress is possibly resolved. Homeostasis begins restoring balance, and a period of recovery enabling repair and renewal takes place. Stress hormone levels may return to normal, but you may have reduced defenses and adaptive energy left as a result. If the stressful condition persists, your body adapts by a continued effort in resistance and remains in a state of arousal. In the third phase, the exhaustion stage, the stress has continued for some time. Your body's ability to resist is lost because its adaptation energy supply is gone. This is sometimes referred to as *overload, burnout, adrenal fatigue,* or *maladaptation.* This stage of the general adaptation syndrome, in which the stress level stays up, is the most hazardous to your health.

Through its ability to adapt to the demands of the environment, the autonomic nervous system plays an essential role in the restoration of balance that gets disrupted by stress. Depending on the stress phase of the person, which can be identified on the person's hands, the reflexologist will know whether the treatment should be based on stimulation of the sympathetic or the parasympathetic nervous system.

The Occipital Zones

The *occiput* is the anatomical term for the posterior (back) portion of the skull. Painfully sensitive to massage when there is a disorder present, the zones of this part of the skull are exact reflections of the structural, sympathetic, or parasympathetic regions that are experiencing the disorder. The painful occipital zones on the head confirm which points on the hand are the ones that require treatment. When treated, a visible state of relaxation results, one that is very helpful to establish before embarking on any further therapeutic reflexology protocol.

Hering's Law

In homeopathy Hering's law is widely recognized as the second law of cure (the first law in homeopathy being "like cures like"). Hering's law, named after Constantine Hering (1800–1880), an early pioneer of homeopathy in the United States, pertains to the direction in which a person's symptoms will disappear during the course of a homeopathic treatment. These are:

▶ from a more important organ to a less important one
▶ from within outward
▶ in the reverse order of the appearance of symptoms
▶ from above downward

My method of total reflexology therapy emphasizes the importance of Hering's law, which the reflexologist can use to follow the evolution or involution of a disease in meticulous detail. Hering's law enables the therapist to monitor the effectiveness of a treatment, to offer the best advice to the patient, and to guide him or her to complementary treatments or medicines.

Hering's Law
Hierarchy of the Symptoms of the Three Levels

MENTAL AND SPIRITUAL BODY

Total mental confusion
Destructive ideas
Paranoid delusions
Delirium, hallucinations
Lethargy
Slow reactions
Dull and absent mind
Lack of concentration
Forgetfulness

EMOTIONAL BODY

Suicidal depression
Apathy
Sorrow
Anger
Fear
Anxiety
Irritability
Lack of satisfaction

PHYSICAL BODY

Brain disorders
Heart problems
Liver problems
Endocrine disorders
Pulmonary disorders
Renal problems
Bone issues
Muscle problems
Skin problems

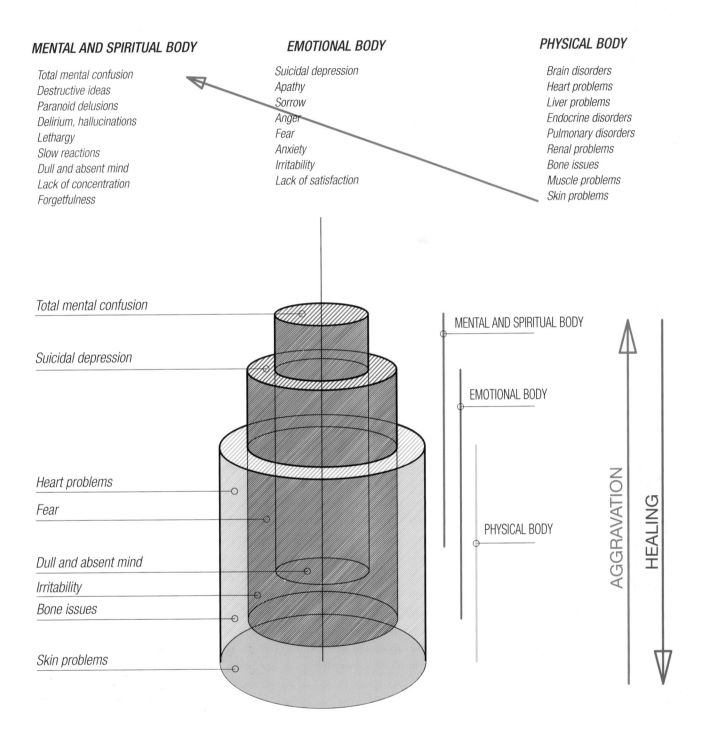

Total mental confusion

Suicidal depression

Heart problems

Fear

Dull and absent mind

Irritability

Bone issues

Skin problems

MENTAL AND SPIRITUAL BODY

EMOTIONAL BODY

PHYSICAL BODY

AGGRAVATION

HEALING

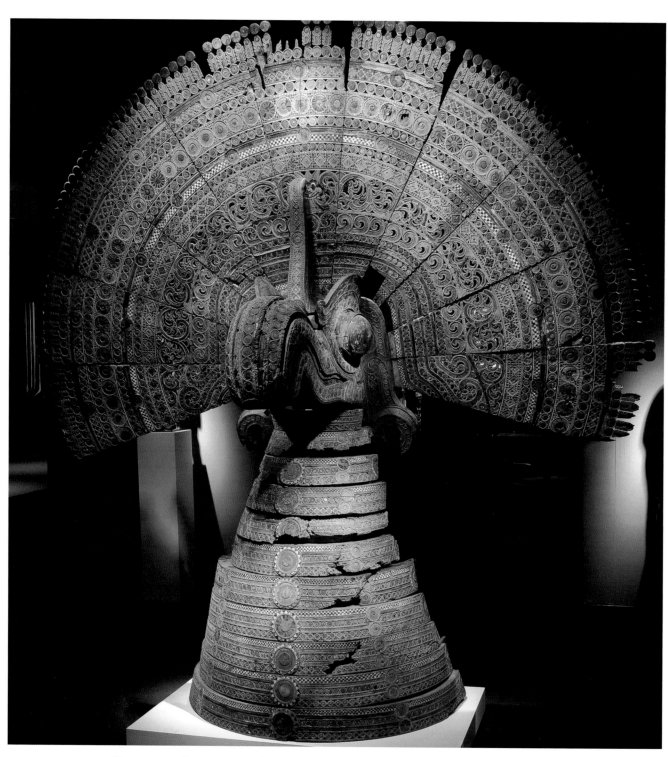

Front part of a processional chariot in wood polychrome from eighteenth-century Kerala, India—an example of the skilled workmanship of the scuulptor made possible by the sensational connection between the hands and the brain

PART TWO

The Sensational Hand-Brain Tandem

The hand is the organ of organs, and the instrument of instruments
for human beings, the active agent of passive powers.

ARISTOTLE

The Hand,
the Servant of the Brain

It is no exaggeration to say that the hands and the brain are inseparable. In fact, to a certain extent the hands are an extension of the brain. Everything that happens in the brain is consistently expressed in the hands. How many things are deemed real if they cannot be touched or seen? How many forms of creative expression and communication are done through the hands? Perceiving is not synonymous with passively receiving an observation originating from the outside; rather, it implies giving an intelligible meaning to such an observation, which often occurs through touch, through the hands. The cerebral cortex of the central region of the brain records the sensitive messages transmitted by touch, and it produces the voluntary, technical movements that are performed by the hands.

The hand is inseparable from human history. In all times, but especially in relatively recent times, we have differentiated between the hands of intellectuals, for example, and those of manual laborers. Superb noble hands or calloused humble hands are emblems of class and trade. Here we will seek to understand how the hands perform so many movements, instruct us in so many events and sensations, acquaint us with what they have learned, and perfectly express our intentions.

The Hand
as a Tool of Human Thought

The human hand is one of the characteristic attributes of our species. It is among the most evolved tools to have served humanity's interests in and requirements for knowledge and evolution. The history of individuals, collectives, ethnic groups, and humanity as a whole is written and transmitted out of the thoughtful maneuvering of a tool by means of the human hand. In this way the distinctiveness of the gestures of the human hand is what separates humanoids from other animals.

The works of humans created by human hands are countless. The abundance, diversity, and magnificence of individual and collective works made by human hands are such that they cause us to forget the importance of human hands throughout civilization. The human hand is the messenger of thought. The Pre-Socratic Greek philosopher Anaxagoras said, "It is because he has hands that man is most intelligent." The anatomical and functional arrangement of the human hand accentuates its abilities to do everything, and therefore its value as a universal tool for touching and grasping. What is extraordinary about the hand is not simply the organ itself as much as everything it enables a person to do with it, from the trivial to the sublime, the futile to the essential, the indispensable to the utilitarian, the superfluous to the useful, and from the horrible to the noble. The hand that chipped the first flint or plucked the first fruit; the hand of the baker kneading dough; the hand of the child learning how to write; the hands of Macbeth and Chopin, and those of Michelangelo painting the hands of Adam's Eternal Father on the ceiling of the Sistine Chapel; the hands of the mountain climber making sure of his hold; the hand of the louse-infested person scratching away at his scalp; and the hands of the sculptor giving shape to a block of stone—these are all hands. The hand provides treatment; the hand heals; the hand transmits energy and vitality. The hand appears as a universal organ of relation and knowledge, of expression and communication, the agent that incorporates reality and executes the individual thought. The realization of ideas and feelings is made concrete with the hands. The hand of a human being is a machine with countless possibilities. No other organ executes the needs, requirements, desires, and wishes with such availability, consistency, exactitude, and loyalty.

The Anatomy of the Hand

The anatomical study of the hand goes back as far as the second-century Greek physician Galen, probably the most accomplished medical researcher of antiquity, who influenced the development of anatomy, physiology, pathology, pharmacology, and neurology, in addition to studying philosophy and logic. However, understanding of the physiology of the hand's movements only began with the nineteenth-century French neurologist Duchenne de Boulogne. Even today, despite the plethora of neurophysiological investigations of the hand, there are still some hazy areas surrounding certain details of its functional anatomy.

In reflexology, to better determine the precise location of which reflex points to stimulate, it is important to first have some basic knowledge of the bones of the hand.

The hand is part of the upper limb, the arm, allowing it maximum efficacy for performing actions. It inserts itself into three-dimensional space in a precise direction and at a given distance. The proper positioning of the hand—appropriate height, distance, and depth—is governed by the conjugal action of the arm and forearm moved by the muscles of the shoulder and elbow. *Supination* describes the movement of the hand and forearm in which the radius turns laterally around its longitudinal axis with the palm facing up. The reverse movement is called *pronation,* in which the palm faces down.

The hand consists of three parts: the wrist, the palm, and the five fingers. Furthermore, there are three kinds of joints: the hinge joints in the articulations of the four fingers, which function like the hinges of a door as they "open and close" on one plane; the arthrodial joints located between the bones of the wrist, only allow a lesser range of movements—small sacks, or bursa, located between the joints, allow the bones to glide easily over each other; the saddle joints are a unique characteristic of the thumb and provide more flexibility than a hinge or gliding joint.

The first row of carpal bones, the assembly that connects the hand to the forearm, forms, by means of the group of the posterior surfaces of the first three bones, an articular surface that fits into the corresponding hollow at the anterior portion of the radius. The hand has at least twenty-seven bones that are joined together or connected to the forearm by twenty-eight joints.

The carpus (wrist) consists of eight bones, in two rows of four. They are all connected to the bone of the forearm. The first row, from the column of the thumb to the fifth finger, consists of

▶ the scaphoid bone
▶ the lunate bone
▶ the triquetral bone
▶ the pisiform bone

The second row, from the column of the thumb to the fifth finger, consists of

- ▶ the trapezium bone
- ▶ the trapezoid bone
- ▶ the capitate bone
- ▶ the hamate bone, which holds a hook: the hamulus

The metacarpus (palm) contains five bones, one for each finger.

The fingers have fourteen phalanges—two for the thumbs, three for each of the other fingers:

- ▶ the distal phalanx that holds the fingernail
- ▶ the intermediate phalanx
- ▶ the proximal phalanx that connects the finger to the metacarpus

This anatomy of the hand ensures that the fingers and their phalanges have the possibility of going into action to the fullest possible extent, in whatever direction required.

The palm consists of the metacarpal bones, or metacarpus, forming the intermediate part of the skeletal hand, located between the phalanges of the fingers and the carpal bones of the wrist. The four metacarpal bones, despite their small size, are long bones with a diaphysis and two articular ends. They are attached to the carpal bone by their front end, which is almost a cube shape, or to be more precise, they are connected to three of the bones from the second row of the carpus—the trapezoid, capitate, and hamate. This is how the carpal bone and the last four metacarpals form a set whose parts have little mobility with respect to one

another, and are only capable of slight gliding movements that are intended to give the entire group elasticity. This fixed position of the metacarpals, which is so important from a physiological perspective, has but one exception: the fifth finger.

The interdependence of the hand's constituent segments appears in the study of the hand's functional anatomy. It is the conjoined action of the metacarpus and the first finger that gives the thumb its primacy over the other fingers.

The Movement of the Hand

The immobility of the hand at rest is only an illusion; it is the result of the continuous regulation of the tension and length of the muscles in a naturally balanced position. This consistent balance of the tension—"the tone," as it is sometimes described—of each of the hand's muscles when taking and holding a position is automatically guaranteed by reflexes, with no need of any intervention on the part of the consciousness or will, which are individualized creations of the nervous system.

Through a process that is of an electrochemical nature, nerve fibers conduct an electrical flow into the motor end plate (the ending of a motor nerve fiber in relation to a skeletal muscle fiber) to induce the phenomenon of muscle contraction. In this way, the muscle and its motor nerve form an anatomical functional unity.

The paths leading to the proximity of each muscle are three nerves: the median, the cubital, and the radial. These three nerves share the duty of innervating all the muscles animating all the segments of the hand, with no wasted effort.

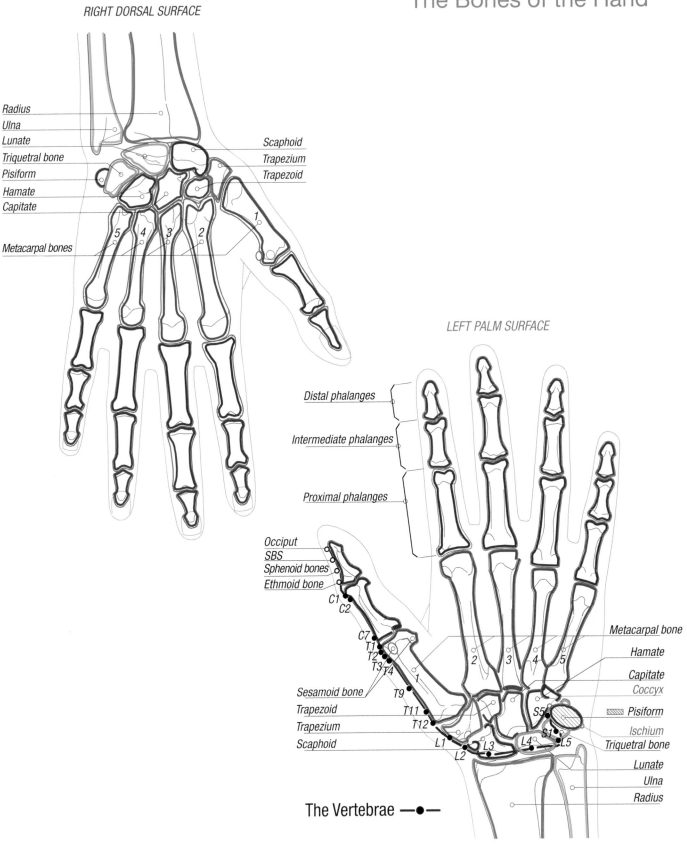

RIGHT DORSAL SURFACE

Radius
Ulna
Lunate
Triquetral bone
Pisiform
Hamate
Capitate

Scaphoid
Trapezium
Trapezoid

Metacarpal bones

5 4 3 2 1

LEFT PALM SURFACE

Distal phalanges

Intermediate phalanges

Proximal phalanges

Occiput
SBS
Sphenoid bones
Ethmoid bone

C1
C2

C7
T1
T2
T3 T4

Sesamoid bone
Trapezoid
Trapezium
Scaphoid

T9

T11
T12

L1
L2
L3

1

2 3 4 5

S5

L4
S1 L5

Metacarpal bone
Hamate
Capitate
Coccyx
Pisiform
Ischium
Triquetral bone
Lunate
Ulna
Radius

The Vertebrae —●—

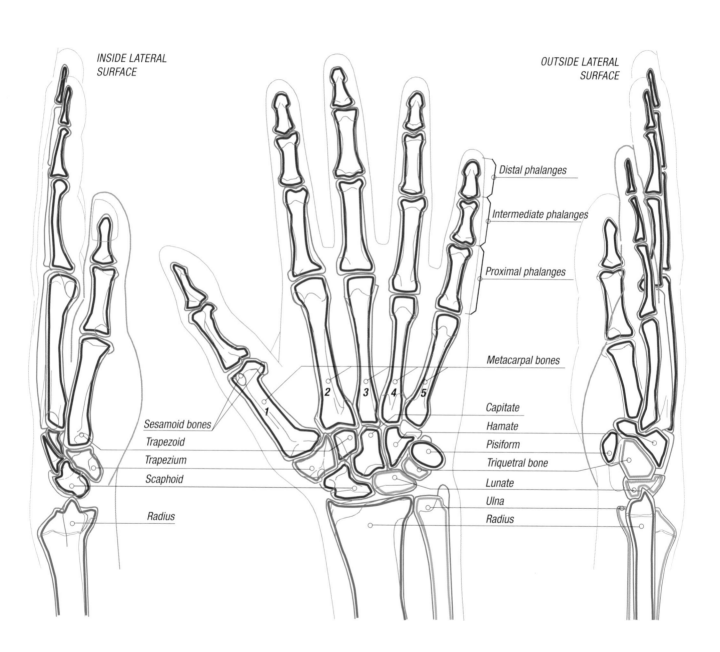

INSIDE LATERAL
SURFACE

OUTSIDE LATERAL
SURFACE

Distal phalanges

Intermediate phalanges

Proximal phalanges

Metacarpal bones

1 2 3 4 5

Sesamoid bones
Trapezoid
Trapezium
Scaphoid

Radius

Capitate
Hamate
Pisiform
Triquetral bone
Lunate
Ulna
Radius

The Spinal Column and Hand Reflex Points

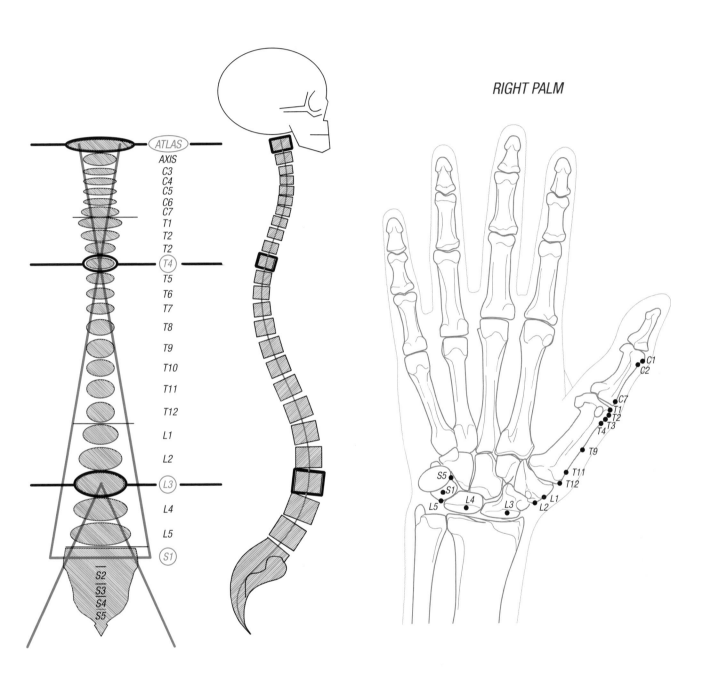

RIGHT PALM

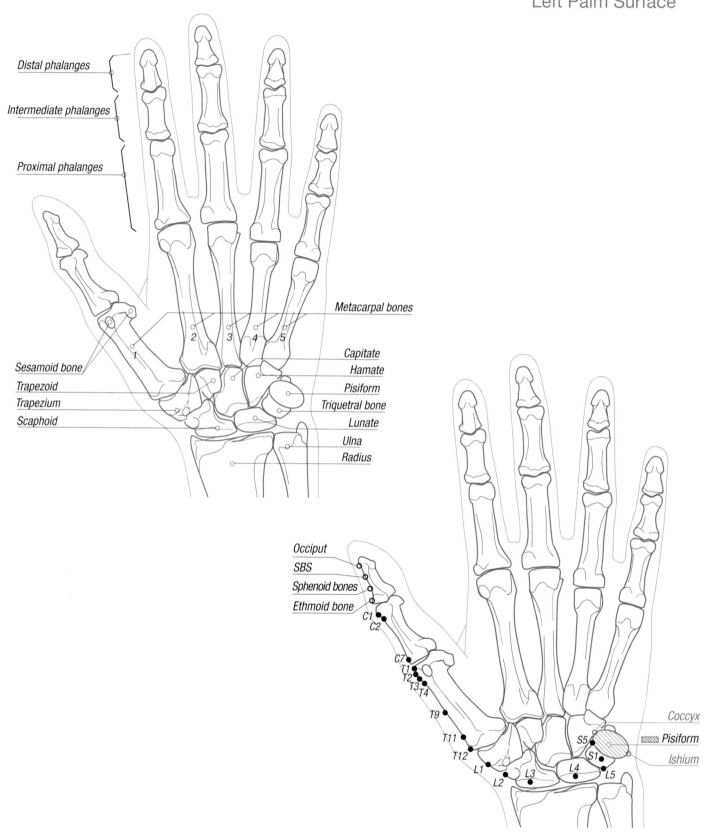

Distal phalanges

Intermediate phalanges

Proximal phalanges

Metacarpal bones

1 2 3 4 5

Sesamoid bone

Trapezoid

Trapezium

Scaphoid

Capitate

Hamate

Pisiform

Triquetral bone

Lunate

Ulna

Radius

Occiput

SBS

Sphenoid bones

Ethmoid bone

C1
C2

C7
T1
T2
T3 T4

T9

T11

T12

L1

L2 L3

L4

S5

S1

L5

Coccyx

Pisiform

Ishium

The Brain,
the Hand's "Motor"

The human being is a vertical biped whose cerebral volume is substantial, hence this distinguishing feature. Aristotle considered vertical posture as one of the essential arrangements that marked the superiority of humans over other animal species. Louis-Jean-Marie Daubenton, an eighteenth-century French naturalist, was the first to make a decisive argument in support of this theory by pointing out the very singular position occupied by the occipital cavity in human beings. Placed beneath the skull instead of opening to the back, it is oriented horizontally, not obliquely. Because of this, the spinal column forms a right angle with the axis of the brain. This arrangement, added to the series of opposing curves of the spinal column, has permitted humans to walk upright, therefore leaving their hands free.

The central sulcus (which is also called the fissure of Rolando, or Rolandic cortex) is the large, deep groove or indentation in the brain that separates the parietal and the frontal lobes and the primary motor cortex from the primary somatosensory cortex. It serves as a general sensorimotor center of integration of the physical regions that are represented there, which include the zones corresponding to the hands, as well as to the mouth and the upper limbs. It is in this area, over the postcentral gyrus, or upper parietal lobe, that we find a topography that corresponds to the shape of our body (the clinical term used is *somatotopic arrangement*). This part of the brain is the point-for-point correspondence of an area of the body to a specific point on the central nervous system. Areas such as the appendages, digits, penis, and face can draw their sensory locations on the somatosensory cortex. The areas that are finely controlled (e.g., the fingers) have larger portions of the somatosensory cortex, whereas areas that are coarsely controlled (e.g., the trunk) have smaller portions. In this way, the overall sensing ability of the body is projected at the level of the parietal lobe of the cerebral cortex, behind the central sulcus, the central fissure.

The fingers and head have a substantial number of sensory receptors and are represented for the most part by peripheral receptors. This is how we build a sensory homunculus, a physical representation of the human body's sensory organs located within the brain. We have approximately one hundred nerve endings at the ends of our fingers that are stimulated by pressure, and around ten thousand neurons that respond to this stimuli. The pressure the fingers make when touching something is most intense at the center point of the thrust, waning and fading toward the sides, and this is recorded in the cortex in the same way.

Qualitative differences apart, from a sensory perspective both humans and apes possess the same

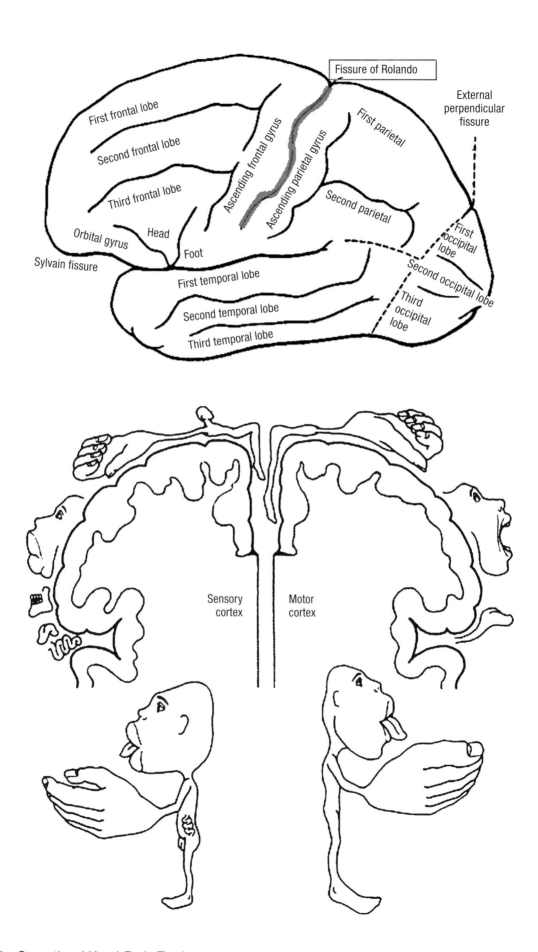

First frontal lobe

Second frontal lobe

Third frontal lobe

Orbital gyrus   Head

Sylvain fissure

Foot

Ascending frontal gyrus

Ascending parietal gyrus

Fissure of Rolando

First parietal

External perpendicular fissure

Second parietal

First occipital lobe

Second occipital lobe

Third occipital lobe

First temporal lobe

Second temporal lobe

Third temporal lobe

Sensory cortex

Motor cortex

neurological potential for facial movements and hand movements with respect to locomotion, gripping ability, food preparation, manipulation, gesticulation, mastication, sucking, swallowing, shouting, mimicry, attacking, and defense. In both species there is a perfect reciprocity between the brain and the hand when it comes to sensory-motor memorization.

The Physiology of the Brain

The brain is an organ that serves as the center of the nervous system in all vertebrates and most inverte-brates. In humans it is the inseparable link between the body and the mind, the relay system between the cosmos and the reality of our body. The biological rhythms that unconsciously govern the individual human being must travel through the brain before initiating bodily function.

The brain weighs about three pounds, which is about 2 percent of total body weight. It consumes 20 percent of the oxygen that is inhaled and uses 60 percent of the carbohydrates taken in by adults (75 percent for a nursing child). There are between 60 to 100 billion cells in the human brain. Each one contains

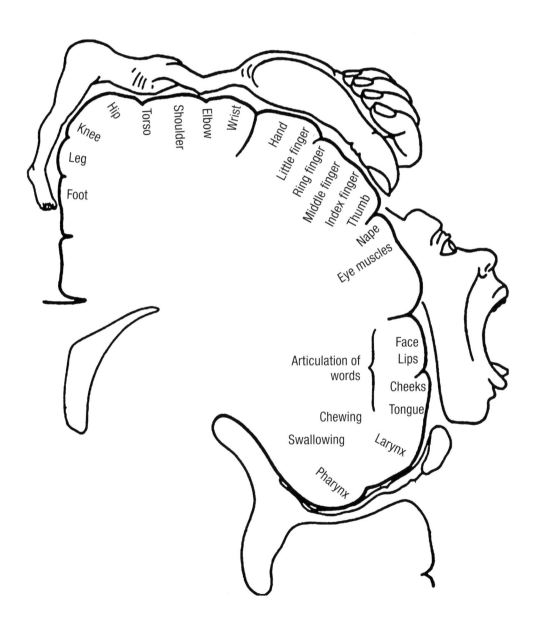

extensions that branch out to form connections with the identical synaptic ends of thousands of other cells. The combinations of cellular groups extend into different zones that have a specific specialty. Because of this, the human brain is extremely complex. It experiences states of awareness that generate pieces of information and impulses, and the stimulations of neurotransmitters.

Cerebral wiring is not a uniform process; it is carried out in accordance with the sensory stimulations that occur during the first weeks and years of childhood, hence the importance of the contact given to the baby vocally, as well as through touch and attention. The circuits of our brain hemispheres are altered through contact with our fellow humans and through our activities until we reach a fairly advanced age. For example, the areas of the cerebral hemispheres corresponding to the hands are much larger in the brain of a sculptor than they are in the brain of a soccer player. This ability of the brain to organize itself in accord with the stimulations it receives does not vanish with the onset of adulthood, and the circuits that offer replacements for this or that function are constantly changing.

The left brain specializes in language as well as logic, rational thinking, calculation, and positive reactions like joy and laughter. The right brain specializes in the hearing of music, intuition, imagination, artistic creation, and spatial orientation.

The Essential Regions of the Brain

Different regions of the brain are at work in the production of conscious experiences, although none of them are capable of maintaining awareness by themselves. If one of these regions is seriously hurt, consciousness will be compromised, altered, or lost. These regions of the brain include:

- supplementary motor area
- motor cortex
- primary visual cortex

- temporal parietal junction
- temporal lobe
- orbitofrontal cortex
- dersolateral prefrontal cortex
- thalamus
- hippocampus
- reticular formation
- cerebellum

Twelve pairs of cranial nerves—nerves that emerge indirectly from the brain (including the brainstem), in contrast to spinal nerves (which emerge from segments of the spinal cord)—originate in the brain. They are essential for a person's relationship to his or her environment. They include:

1. olfactory/gustatory nerve	sensory
2. optic nerve	sensory
3. oculomotor nerve	motor
4. pathetic or trochlear nerve	motor
5. trigeminal nerve	motor/sensory
6. abducens nerve	motor/sensory
7. facial nerve	motor/sensory
8. auditory nerve	sensory
9. glossopharyngeal nerve	motor/sensory
10. pneumogastric or vagus nerve	motor/sensory
11. spinal nerve	motor
12. hypoglossal nerve	motor

Brain Genetics

A gene is a unit of hereditary information comprised of DNA that determines one or more physical characteristics, such as eye color. Its activity relies on the production of proteins. Like switches, genes can adjust their

Reflex Zones of the Cranial Nerves

RIGHT PALM SURFACE

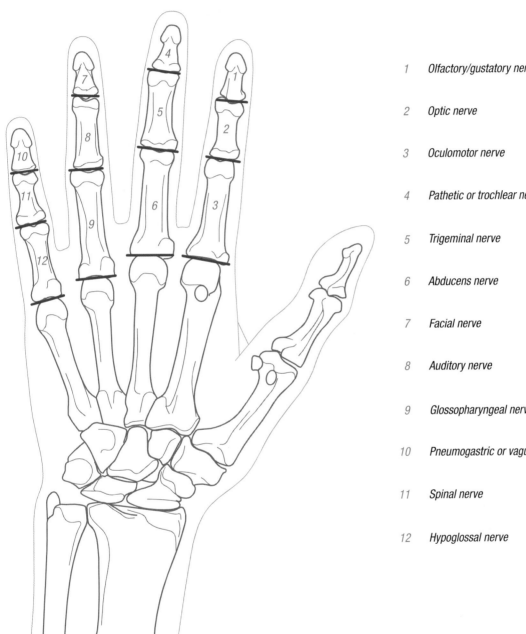

1	Olfactory/gustatory nerve	*sensory*
2	Optic nerve	*sensory*
3	Oculomotor nerve	*motor*
4	Pathetic or trochlear nerve	*motor*
5	Trigeminal nerve	*motor/sensory*
6	Abducens nerve	*motor/sensory*
7	Facial nerve	*motor/sensory*
8	Auditory nerve	*sensory*
9	Glossopharyngeal nerve	*motor/sensory*
10	Pneumogastric or vagus nerve	*motor/sensory*
11	Spinal nerve	*motor*
12	Hypoglossal nerve	*motor*

activity, known as their *expression*. Gene expression in the brain can alter neurotransmitter rate, which in turn will have an effect on complex functions like personality, memory, and intelligence. However, neurotransmitters also have an effect on genetic expression. As well, environmental influences have consequences for the patterns of genetic expression, which is why mental functions also depend on factors like diet, geography, the social network, and the level of stress.

Proteins come into play at different levels in the physiological organism. Some form structures such as hair; others—enzymes produced by the various glands and organs, for example—regulate processes. Some genes of the genome can encode the proteinic molecules that manufacture serotonin, the neurotransmitter at work in moods. Each variation produces a slightly different proteinic molecule of varying effectiveness. This is how genetic variants can cause higher serotonin rates in one person and lower rates in another. A lower rate of serotonin is synonymous with a predisposition for depression or bulimia. This is equally true for other neurotransmitters like dopamine. Dopamine deficiency has been linked to an increased level of risky behaviors such as addiction to alcohol or drugs. This is how our genotype effects brain structure and function, which in turn has an influence on our behavior.

The Sexual Brain

The brains of men and women display differences in terms of structure and function; notably, the corpus callosum and anterior commissure (the original connection between the two cerebral hemispheres that links the regions of the unconscious) are larger in women. This could explain why female emotional consciousness is more developed: the right side of the brain that is connected with emotion has a better connection to the more analytical left side and can also allow emotions to be integrated more easily into thoughts and speech. When performing difficult tasks, women

use both hemispheres, whereas in men, only the hemisphere best suited to the task at hand is called on.

The Developing Brain

In the days following conception, the embryo is a tiny mass of cells. Formation of the brain and nervous system begins at the end of around three weeks with the differentiation of the cells that have just constructed the neural plate in the embryo's back. This plate will expand and fold to form the fluid-filled neural tube, which is the source of the brain and spinal cord. The brain makes its appearance after four weeks in the form of a small bulb at the upper end of the neural tube. Meanwhile the spinal cord gradually takes shape at the other end of this tube, with all of this coming from the ectoderm. The main parts of the brain such as the cortex are visible starting around the seventh week.

Around the age of five, the human hippocampus reaches maturity and allows the formation of memories. Before this time very few memories can be stored away. At around the age of seven, the axons of the reticular formation of the brain stem are covered by a myelin sheath, which allows an increased ability to pay attention. Growth spurts between the ages of six and fifteen trigger the transformation of the regions that are at play in language and the understanding of spatial relations, mainly in the parietal lobe. These changes are intimately linked to intellectual and social development, such as the ability to read and make friends.

The parietal and temporal lobes connected with the spatial, sensorial, auditory, and language-related areas of the brain reach maturity in adolescence. The brain is then ready to meet a number of social and intellectual challenges. However, the prefrontal cortex, whose involvement in thinking and planning is essential, is still developing. This is why it seems that the treatment of emotional information in adolescents is especially reliant on the amygdala, the two almond-shaped groups of nuclei located deep and medially within the temporal lobes of the brain that perform a primary role in the processing of memory, decision making, and emotional reactions. This could explain adolescents' seeming lack of good judgment and their mood swings.

The activity patterns of the adult brain reflect their emotional maturity. The treatment of emotional information activates the frontal lobe more intensely in the adult brain than in that of the adolescent, which leads to perceptions that have been more thought out. The prefrontal cortex that is associated with the ability to examine the consequences of one's actions and general reasoning abilities is the last region of the brain to reach maturity. The hippocampus is one of the only parts of the brain capable of producing neurons in adulthood, but the significance of this phenomenon has yet to be made fully clear.

The Aging Brain

Old age is generally associated with the decline of both the body and the mind, which is true to the extent that we lose neurons at this stage of life and those that remain transmit impulses more slowly. This causes delays in the thinking process, creates memory problems, and causes deterioration of the reflexes, which in turn induces problems of balance and movement. Most neurons remain healthy until death, but the size and volume of the brain shrinks from 5 to 10 percent between the ages of twenty and ninety. The myelin sheath that covers the axons of the neurons is essential for effective transmission between the cells. This protein-based structure wears down with age, causing the cerebral circuits to be less effective and causing problems with balance and memory. In addition, studies have shown that dopamine, the neurotransmitter that is at work in creating arousal and making quick decisions, diminishes with age. This brings about behavioral changes, as dopamine is linked to strong sensations and taking risks. This explains why elderly people prefer a calm and quiet life.

There is, however, an upside to aging from the standpoint of brain function. The brain understands the effects of aging, and certain mental functions can even improve with age. The increase of the myelin of the frontal and temporal lobes between the ages of forty and fifty make it easier to manage what one knows. Furthermore, studies on comprehension show that older people use high-level functions that are served by both hemispheres, or that of a different hemisphere than those more inferior levels utilized by younger adults. This is how the brain makes up for the loss of function in order for the processes of memory and thinking to remain sharp.

What is more, new studies on aging reveal that the decline of cerebral function can be slowed down by a number of lifestyle factors. For example, it has been shown that eating less ensures lower blood sugar levels, which can slow the appearance of changes because glycemia causes damage to proteins. People with high blood sugar such as those with type 1 diabetes show more signs of aging in the brain than nondiabetic persons. Other factors connected to lifestyle can actually stimulate the growth of neuronal tissue in old age. Moderate physical exercise such as power walking, regular sleep, a good diet, and brain exercises can delay the decline of cerebral function and provide protection against problems inherent to aging, such as memory loss.

Consciousness

How do the electrical discharges of the cerebral cells generate our conscious experience of the world and thereby our sense of self and our capacity for abstract thought? Answering this question requires an understanding of the bridge between the physical and the mental worlds. As research in the neurosciences progresses, we can begin to gain a better understanding of what consciousness is and how it is produced. This is how a correlation can be established between different states of consciousness and the activity of clearly defined cerebral regions.

But what exactly is consciousness? Consciousness refers to our mind and thoughts, to the normal state of being awake and aware. We know that consciousness is essential, that life would have no meaning without it. We are capable of identifying the kinds of activities that produce consciousness, but the way this a priori, intangible phenomenon arises out of a physical organism remains something of a mystery. There is nothing comparable to consciousness. A thought, sensation, or idea seems to be different from the material objects that comprise the rest of the world. The contents of our mind cannot be situated in time or space. Although consciousness appears to be produced by particular kinds of physical activities in the brain, we do not know if these activities form part of consciousness itself, or if cerebral activity is a correlation with different elements that together comprise consciousness. And while consciousness is not restricted to cerebral activity, it still correlates with these various elements that form the mind, or awareness, when they work together. This suggests that the material universe is simply one aspect of reality, and that consciousness is a kind of parallel reality in which entirely different rules apply.

Consciousness appears to arise in three stages: (1) the data related to visual stimuli enters the brain; (2) this data generates cerebral activity; and (3) this cerebral activity allows the mind to have conscious perception. Thus human consciousness is the result of the interaction of different parts of the body with its environment. The brain plays a crucial role in the production of waking consciousness but we still do not know why some processes inside the brain and the neuronal activity of different regions establish a solid correlation with consciousness, whereas others do not. These processes and regions appear to be necessary for the production of consciousness, although they are insufficient to produce it on their own.

Levels and Types of Consciousness

Consciousness is expressed through a variety of modes such as emotions, sensations, thoughts, and perceptions, all felt at different levels of neuronal activity, attention, and concentration. The level of neuronal activity determines the intensity of consciousness. Attention can be turned toward the outside world or toward the inner one (musing over one's thoughts). Concentration can be lightly focused, directed toward different objects, or solidly targeting a specific aspect. *Concentration* is the term used to express one-pointed focus on an object; this kind of attention allows one to overlook other focal points.

A distinction is made between three kinds of consciousness: that of the present moment, in which the brain takes in events as they occur and reacts, but these occurrences are not transcribed into the memory; waking consciousness, in which events are recorded and transcribed into memory; and self-consciousness, in which events are recorded, coded into memory, and recalled, such that the person is conscious of what he or she is doing. Different types of neuronal activity in the brain are associated with waking consciousness. The neuronal activity of the cortex, particularly that of the frontal lobe, is combined with the appearance of conscious experience. A stimulus taken in by the brain becomes conscious in half a second. The neuronal activity triggered by the stimulus occurs first in the lower reaches of the brain, such as the amygdala and thalamus, before reaching the upper regions in the parts of the cortex that deal with sensations. As a general rule, the frontal cortex is only active when an experience becomes conscious, which suggests that its involvement is an essential element of consciousness.

Memory

Memory, as an aspect of consciousness, is the power or process of reproducing or recalling what has been learned and retained, especially through associative mechanisms. Even though we quickly forget most of the moments we experience, some remain stored in the brain in the form of memories. When we remember something, the neurons involved with the event that created this memory are activated. Memories, however, are simply reconstructions of the past and not its repetition, as their primary purpose is to provide us with information that can guide our present actions.

Physiologically, memory refers to a certain number of cerebral functions whose common characteristic is to recreate past experiences by synchronizing the discharge of neurons involved in the original experience. Memory encompasses a large field of aspects and functions, extending from the instincts that are most deeply rooted, to conscious factual knowledge, with all these different elements of memory associated with different regions of the brain. Frontal lobe activity guarantees that memories conform to reality. Episodic memories are activated in those regions of the brain with the experience we wish to recall. The hippocampus is the region where events are converted into memories.

Love and Attachment

Where do our feelings of love and attachment to others, which are expressions of consciousness, come from? Oxytocin is a hormone produced by the hypothalamus. It is released by the stimulation of the sexual and reproductive organs during orgasm and birth. It creates a sense of well-being and encourages the formation of attachments with others, most likely because in parallel with vasopressin, to which it is closely connected, it contributes to the processing of social indexes involved in the recognition of people; for this reason it may also play a role in the construction of common memories. It is possible that oxytocin, like dopamine, creates a feeling of dependency, which would explain why people feel anxiety at the thought of being away from those they love; the absence of the rise of oxytocin that is felt in the presence of the beloved is perceived as something missing.

Kissing, hugging, and cuddling releases oxytocin into the bloodstream, which intensifies feelings of intimacy and strengthens the bonds between partners. Human beings form attachments—bonds of intimacy and affection—to people, animals, and objects. Just how important these attachments are became evident during the two world wars, when babies in orphanages were observed over time. Though housed and fed, these babies did not have the protection or care assured by a parent. This caused children to become incapable of forming bonds of friendship or even love after they reached adulthood.

Sleeping and Dreaming

We spend close to a third of our life sleeping, a period during which the brain remains active to ensure that multiple functions continue to run smoothly. The brain manufactures dreams, which are sometimes the source of some strange and intense experiences. No one knows exactly why sleep is so important. Common thinking is that it provides a time of rest during which the body can "auto-prepare" itself. It gives us an opportunity to remain relatively safe from danger and in a calm, stress-free state for a portion of the day. It is also hypothesized that the brain needs to disconnect from the outside world so it can sort through, deal with, and commit to memory information received while awake. What is indisputable is that sleep is essential for our health. If we do not get enough sleep, our ability to think and remember things clearly will rapidly diminish.

There is no doubt that some functions concerning memory occur during sleep, but we have no absolute certainty that these are necessary. The cycles of sleeping and waking are controlled by neurotransmitters that act on the brain to trigger various phases. Studies suggest that a chemical substance called *adenosine,* which is present in the blood, is what provokes the desire to fall asleep, and its effects dissipate while we are sleeping. Located in the hypothalamus, the ventrolateral preoptic nucleus manufactures y-aminobutyric acid

(GABA), a neurotransmitter that spreads into the waking centers and deactivates them so that we can sleep.

Selfhood

A sense of our own selfhood is the a priori condition of our consciousness. It presents itself in various forms, and it steps in at different levels of our consciousness.

The human brain generates an idea of the self that permits us to appropriate our experiences and establish a connection between our thoughts and intentions, and our body and our actions. Our sense of self allows us to analyze our mind and use what we see to guide our behavior. The physical self is transcribed onto different mental "maps" on which our experiences are recorded. The more fragile mental self is closely connected with the ability to find our personal memories. In short, to be aware, the brain must appropriate its perceptions—in other words, it must recognize that they are occurring within the person's mind. To do this, we must generate a sense of self.

The Cranial Concept

Applying the cranial concept to reflexology is of fundamental importance because of the large number of people suffering from injuries connected to cranial trauma, which causes structural damage. In the majority of cases, this trauma can be traced back to birth. For example, after Dr. Viola Frymann examined 1,250 newborns (as described in her 1966 book, *Disturbances of the Cranio Sacral Mechanisms*), she only found that 11.6 percent did not exhibit any deformation. Pediatric problems, migraines, sterility, and the degeneration of old age, especially, can all be treated through cranial therapy. As well, many psychiatric disorders can be traced to one or more traumas affecting the occipital-mastoid region, the sphenobasilar symphysis (*the articulation of the sphenoid with the occiput), or* the fronto-ethmoidal and ethmoidal articulations.

Understanding the craniosacral system is preliminary to understanding the relationships that exist between the nervous, skeletal-muscular, vascular, lymphatic, endocrine, and respiratory systems (as described in detail in part 4). Any disruption in these systems can have an influence on the craniosacral region and the functioning of the brain and spinal cord. To understand the craniosacral system and how a craniosacral treatment works, it is important to know the broad architecture of the parts of the body involved.

The Bony Structures

The sphenoid bone is the butterfly-shaped bone of the neurocranium, situated in the middle of the skull toward the front, in front of the temporal bone and basilar part of the occipital bone. At around the age of eleven the sphenoid bone articulates, and by the twenty-fifth year the sphenoid and occipital are completely fused.

The sphenoid is of major importance in the mobility of the cranial base, vault, and face. Ocular migraines are most often caused by membranous tensions on the greater wing of the sphenoid bone that affect the sphenobasilar symphysis and involving the sphenoidal fissure, which in turn affects the cranial nerves that travel through it. These nerves influence the muscles and intentional movements of the eye, which in this case leads to contractions and sharp pain in this area. Reflex massage of the cranial zones of the feet or hands restores the exchange of fluids across the body, eliminates stasis in traumatized tissues, and thereby restores biochemical and bioelectrical balance.

At the base of the skull, between the sphenoid bone and the occiput, we find the sphenobasilar symphysis. Semimobile, it constitutes the only true articulation of the skull. Located within its center, it transmits to the bones of the skull its rhythmic movement of contraction and expansion, which it receives from the fluids provided by the ventricular system of the brain.

There are three groupings of twenty-nine bones of

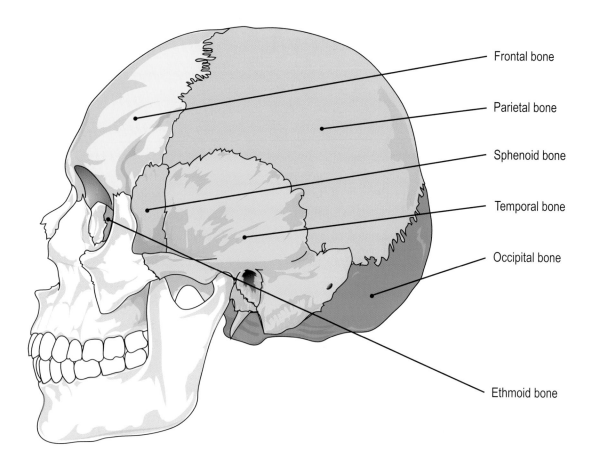

Frontal bone

Parietal bone

Sphenoid bone

Temporal bone

Occipital bone

Ethmoid bone

the skull articulated in the movements of flexion, extension, and rotation, which are transmitted down the spinal column to the bones of the sacrum, and from there descending through the legs, arms, hands, and feet.

▶ The **cranial base** is formed from the frontal bone, the ethmoid bone, the bulk of the sphenoid bone, the petrous part of the temporal bone, the condyle portion at the base of the occiput, and the sphenobasilar symphysis; it facilitates the movement of flexion and extension.

▶ The **cranial vault** consists of the frontal bone, the ethmoid bone, the two parietal bones, the sphenoid bone and its lateral wings, the two temporal bones, and the occiput.

▶ The **nucleus** or **spinal column** (i.e., core link) consists of a tube containing the three meninges that connects the sacrum to the occipital cavity. This membrane is fairly free inside the spinal channel and is only attached at the second sacral vertebra.

The Membranes

The fasciae and the meninges are the primary membranes of the body.

The fasciae are the fibers of connective tissue (mainly collagen) that travel between the viscera, nerves, and blood vessels, and envelop all the organs. They support the bones and connect the muscular tissues and connective tissues of the body. They have an influence on circulation and the drainage of the wrapped organs, and because of this they are of great importance for their vitality. They are stimulated or regulated by the nervous system, and directly relate to the craniosacral system and its movement.

The meninges are brain sheaths; there are three types:

▶ The **dura mater** is the outside layer that envelops the brain and spinal cord. Its hard and nonelastic connective tissue is attached to the bone of the skull by vertical bands (the falx of the cerebrum and the falx of the cerebellum) and a horizontal membrane (the tentorium) (see page 34).

▶ The **arachnoid** is extremely delicate and highly vascularized. It is separated from the dura mater and the pia mater by the subarachnoid space, which is filled with cerebrospinal fluid. Because of its flexibility it permits a more independent movement than that of the other meninges.

▶ The **pia mater** is closely attached to the brain to whose circumvolutions it adheres, then runs along the spinal cord on into the spinal column, thereby assuring its independence of movement.

Cerebrospinal Fluid

The volume held by the brain and spinal cord together is around 56 fluid ounces, of which a little more than five ounces is taken up by cerebrospinal fluid (CSF). This fluid is contained within the brain's ventricles, in the cisterns located around and beneath the brain, and in the subarachnoidal space. It travels from the brain down the spinal column and spinal cord until it finally meets the sacrum. All of these containers act as protectors of the fluids for the central nervous system.

The American osteopathic physician William Sutherland (1873–1954) was among the first in the biological domain to recognize the interchangeability of energy and matter (which forms Einstein's famous formula $E = MC^2$). The cerebrospinal fluid has its own intelligence; in dynamic relationship with the physiological function of every cell of the body, it is, in certain respects, the "breath of life," an electrical potential that charges and discharges itself through its substance and its sphere of influence. Sutherland had the brilliance to use the intelligence of this "liquid light" to diagnose and correct cranial lesions affecting the brain's membranes and articulations; he was the first osteopathic physician to conceptualize the cranial approach and teach it systematically.

Several recent discoveries in atomic medicine have shed light on what Sutherland put into practice. Nuclear physics makes it possible to understand what cerebrospinal fluid is: a vital mechanism that has a powerful influence on human physiology. Considered the most evolved element of the body, CSF performs numerous essential functions. It

▶ nourishes the cerebral cells

▶ bathes the exterior of the central nervous system and contributes to its metabolism

▶ protects the brain from shocks

▶ transmits the vibration of the pituitary and pineal glands, carrying their hormones into the bloodstream, which then transports them to the cells' receptors

▶ transports the hormonal secretions of the pituitary gland's posterior lobe

▶ transmits the flexion and extension rhythm of the craniosacral mechanism

▶ guarantees the protection and energetic restoration of the body

The Anatomy of Cerebrospinal Fluid

CSF is manufactured by the choroid plexuses in the lateral spaces, and in the third and fourth ventricles that act as shock absorbers around the brain. Five fluid

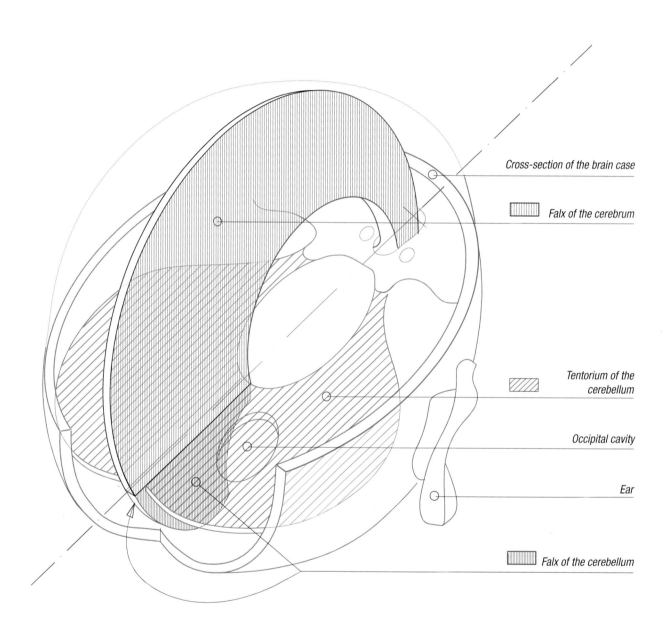

Cross-section of the brain case

Falx of the cerebrum

Tentorium of the cerebellum

Occipital cavity

Ear

Falx of the cerebellum

ounces of CSF transmit the pulsations of the brain; they enter the nerves and connective tissues and supply information, stimulation, and nourishment.

CSF is regulated at a level of constant pressure. In this way it serves as a shock absorber for the brain inside the brain case. Any change in its fluctuation is an indication of a disorder. Through its activity of distribution, nutrition, and cleansing of the nerve cells, the cerebrospinal fluid nourishes all the structures of the brain and spinal cord. In this capacity it

- acts as a filter and vacuum cleaner
- transports hormones and peptides
- serves as a fluid protector of the brain, finding balance with other bodily fluids such as blood and lymph
- influences the primary respiratory mechanism (PRM) or cerebral breathing through its pH and, indirectly, influences pulmonary respiration (if too acidic, physiological cellular exchanges will not take place)
- serves as a chemical and physical agent of protection and consequently helps in the transmission of the cells' nervous, emotional, and mental impulses

The Primary Respiratory Mechanism

William Sutherland discovered and named what is known as the *primary respiratory mechanism* (PRM), a central premise of craniosacral therapy. This term is used in conjunction with the therapist's manipulation of the synarthrodial joints of the cranium and the application of light touches to the patient's spine and pelvis, thereby regulating the flow of cerebrospinal fluid. In this way we can see a rhythmic movement (bending and extending) made up of the movement of the sutures that articulate the twenty-nine bones of the cranial vault. The articular mobility of the skull permits the brain to expand and contract. This depends on

- the fluctuations of the cerebrospinal fluid
- the connections of the tentorium and the falx of the cerebrum
- the contacts of the pituitary gland in the sella turcica
- the frontal lobes in the anterior cranial fossa
- the temporal lobes in the middle cranial fossa against the squama temporalis
- the greater wings of the sphenoid bone
- the contacts of the cerebellum against the squama occipitalis

The rhythm of the PRM can be perceived throughout the body. It is important to know how to recognize its quality and intensity (see page 51 for more on assessing the PRM); a low range means the presence of weakened energy and a lower resistance to infections. If it displays a lack of symmetry, this can make it possible for pathological problems to be located.

The central nervous system (consisting of the brain and spinal cord) possesses the amazing mobility of a jellyfish, and the fluctuations of craniosacral fluid are in relation to the mobility of the central nervous system. The meninges (or membranes of reciprocal tension) are the agents ensuring the mobility of the cranial and craniosacral mechanisms, helping, restricting, and controlling their movement.

The articular mobility of the sacrum between the iliac bones is involuntary not postural. When breathing in, the movement of the foramen of the skull lifts the dura mater, the central bond between the skull and pelvis, and the connective tissue. This is a movement of flexion and extension of the brain case via the spinal column, the spinal cord, and its membranes.

Homeostasis relies on the PRM, with the central nervous system regulating the voluntary effects and the autonomic nervous system the involuntary ones. Brain function is triggered to receive information by the perception of electromagnetic and sound waves translated into electrical impulses. The cerebrospinal fluid and its movement of flexion and extension are the result of a rhythmic pumping directed by the glial cells of the brain. The cerebrospinal fluid retains a memory of all the electromagnetic information it receives. It transmits this information to the entire body by means of the spinal cord and connective tissue.

The PRM is essential to body and organ function. It can be disrupted in various ways that affect its rhythm, volume, fluctuation rate, and composition. These adverse changes can have a bone origin as a result of structural problems, including those affecting movement or posture; a traumatic origin due to an alteration of the structure of the skull or spinal column; or an intrauterine or natal origin that exhibits in articular-membranous lesions. By working on the skull, the osteopath can guide its movements to liberate the articulations, ligaments, and membranes, while in reflexology the practitioner's hands can accomplish the same thing by means of a highly effective technique that works indirectly on the brain, through the hands or feet.

The Choroid Plexus

The choroid plexus is a plexus of cells that produces the cerebrospinal fluid in the ventricles of the brain. It serves as the kidneys of the brain. CSF flushes four times a day in order to clean out metabolites and toxins like beta amyloid, separating them from the blood that contains nutritious substances, ions, and other essential molecules from the CSF. As a result, the choroid plexus must produce about 500 milliliters of CSF daily. By this flushing mechanism it ensures the chemical stability of the CSF, in which the cells of the brain are immersed with the arachnoid and the cerebral capillary network.

The barrier between the blood and the CSF is a vital one, as there is an exchange of substances with the interstitial fluid that surrounds the neurons and glial cells. The choroid plexus selectively governs the molecular exchanges between the CSF and the blood. A secretor of cerebrospinal fluid, it guarantees it a stable milieu and enriches it with the nutritive substances it extracts from the blood.

Connective Tissue

The organization of the connective tissue into chains of fascia (the superficial aponeurosis; the deep cervical thoracic, abdominal-pelvic chains; and the meninges membranes) that are stretched over the skeleton ensure the interdependent interactions of all parts of the body. The connective tissue, along with the bones, muscles, and fasciae, serves as a stabilizer of the body's equilibrium.

Connective tissue is a reservoir of chemical substances. It supports, connects, and separates different types of tissues and organs in the body, including epithelial, muscle, and nervous tissue. It serves as the body's garbage collector. It forms part of its defense mechanisms and immune system, absorbing and digesting bacteria (phagocytosis), foreign bodies, and the tissues that should be eliminated. The connective tissue is therefore the arena where inflammatory processes take place.

The father of osteopathy, Andrew Taylor Still (1828–1917), said, "The fascia [i.e., the connective tissue] is the place to look for finding the cause of the disease." Every physical trauma or emotional or mental conflict can echo in the muscle tone and posture. Stress bands can be found in the fasciae. For example, a postural defect resulting from an accumulation of fascial and articular muscular tension can cause chronic fatigue. A joint trauma encourages fibrosis, and abnormally extended fasciae will shrink and thicken. The response is hyperemia, followed by congestion, edema, and ischemia. The changes in pressure that this causes can affect the nerves, the blood, and the lymphatic vessels, and can disrupt the stimulation and nutrition of the tissues. In addition to these mechanical factors, food deficiencies, toxins, climactic variations, and so forth can also bring about disruptions in connective tissue function.

In the context of self-healing and self-defense, the vital forces first attempt to repel the adverse forces, and if they are not entirely successful in doing so the body will become stuck in a pattern of adaptation and compensation. These adverse forces will remain ever ready to put in a new appearance. Physical fatigue, a toxic emotion, or a toxic state can relaunch the battle, and all the symptoms associated with it. In this struggle, there can be a loss of energy and freedom caused by the adherence formed between the connective tissue and the neighboring tissues.

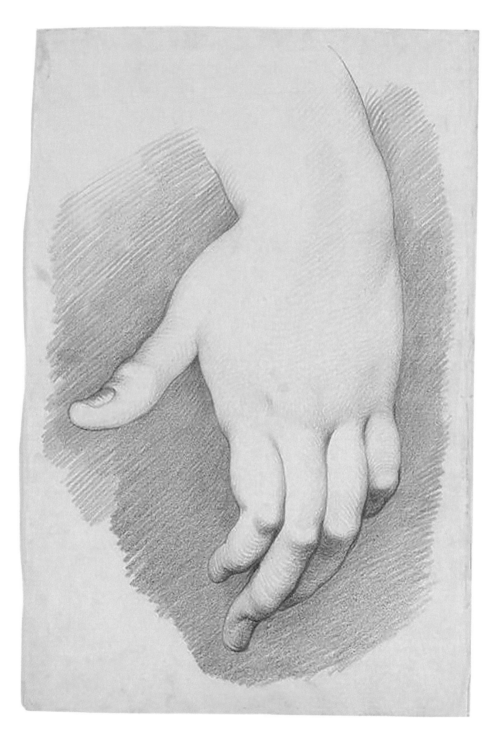

Sanguine, or red chalk, drawing of hand

PART THREE

The Therapeutic Experience

Behold the hands, how they promise, conjure, appeal, menace, pray, supplicate, refuse, beckon, interrogate, admire, confess, cringe, instruct, command, mock and what not besides, with a variation and multiplication of variation which makes the tongue envious.

MICHEL DE MONTAIGNE

The Basics of Reflexology

Hand reflexology treats the diseases that affect organ function as pertains to vascularization (also known as *angiogenesis,* the development of new blood vessels) and innervation (the distribution or supply of nerves to a body part). The effects of reflexology are felt both on the surface and in the depths of the body.

According to principles of naturopathy, reflexology restores cellular balance by improving

► the quality of the intra- and extracellular fluids
► circulation (lymphatic, blood, and cerebrospinal)
► nerve and electromagnetic nutrition

This improvement at the cellular level, with the resulting restored movement of the fluids, has a beneficial effect on all the body's systems: hormonal, nervous, and so on.

Restoring Energy through Therapeutic Touch

With respect to therapeutic touch and its many benefits, we need only note that the "laying on of hands" is a practice that goes back to the dawn of time. Even today in Great Britain, this therapeutic practice is quite widespread in hospitals and palliative-care centers. A reflexology massage provides a sense of well-being that makes it easier to resist the effects of stress and disease. This kind of pleasant physical touch prompts the release of chemical substances called *endomorphins,* which are endogenous opioid peptides that produce pleasure and stimulate the production of T cells that are essential for the functioning of the immune system. Additionally, touch increases the release of melatonin, a hormone whose antidepressant effects play a positive role on mood. In this way reflexology works like an antidepressant medication to chase off sorrow, restore the joy of living, and inspire mental energy.

The notion of the existence of an electromagnetic circuit or meridians, along with the Eastern concept of *chi* (or *qi,* the underlying principle of traditional Chinese medicine, referring to life force or energy flow), are foundational to understanding how energy circulates within the body. As it happens, stress and disease interfere with the transmission of this energy flow. Reflexology, like acupuncture, releases blockages and frees the energetic circuitry, thus restoring to the body its fundamental harmony and equilibrium.

The regions of the body and corresponding reflex points of the hand are:

The phalanxes of the ten fingers: the head and its network of veins and arteries, the cranial nerves, the brain, and the primary sense organs

The metacarpals: the thoracic cavity, including the respiratory tract, the lungs, the heart, and the mediastinum

The carpal bones: the abdominal cavity beneath the

diaphragm, including the digestive tract, stomach, liver, pancreas, spleen, and intestines

The pisiform bone: the pelvic cavity, including the urinary and genital tracts, the lower part of the intestine marked off by the two hips, the sacrum, and the coccyx

The inner edge of the hand: the spinal column, including the autonomic nervous system

Embryological Basics

Embryology, the branch of biology that studies the development of sex cells, fertilization, and development of embryos and fetuses, makes it possible to understand how a skin zone can have a connection to an organ (or a bone or blood vessel, the nervous system, the lymphatic system, certain muscles, or the layers of flat, broad tendons):

▶ The skin and brain are produced out of the ectoderm (the outermost of the three primary layers of an embryo).

▶ The skeleton, soft tissue, and muscles are produced from the mesoderm (the middle of the three primary layers of an embryo).

▶ The digestive tract (from mouth to anus) is produced from the endoderm (the innermost of the three primary layers of an embryo).

The neural tube is the embryo's precursor to the central nervous system, which comprises the brain and spinal cord. It develops in four phases:

Phase 1: Three layers of differentiated cells form the embryonic disk in the amniotic cavity. The neural groove and fold appear in the region of the ectoderm.

Phase 2: The neural folds expand, topped by the neural crest.

Phase 3: The neural folds merge to form the neural tube. The mesoderm seeperates into bone, muscular, and connective tissue. The crescent formed by the endoderm closes up to form a tube.

Phase 4: The skin, digestive tract, neural tube, and intestines are now separate entities. The neural crest emerges as the neural root of the ganglions.

Thus the three embryonic sheets—the ectoderm, mesoderm, and endoderm—develop out of the amniotic cavity and initiate the conduction of the neural pathways that control a reflex action that is illuminated by reflexology. There are two forms of these neural pathways, called *reflex arcs:* monosynaptic and polysynaptic. When a reflex arc consists of only two neurons, it is defined as monosynaptic. So, for example, in the case of peripheral muscle reflexes (e.g., patellar reflex or "knee jerk," and achilles reflex), brief stimulation to the muscle spindle results in contraction of the agonist or effector muscle. By contrast, in polysynaptic reflex pathways, one or more interneurons connect sensory and motor signals. All but the simplest reflexes are polysynaptic, allowing processing or inhibition of polysynaptic reflexes within the brain.

A specific articular, visceral, or muscular zone will respond to a stimulation of the skin by means of a monosynaptic or a polysynaptic reflex arc, and vice versa. The nerve flow originating in the marrow will reach the surface, conveying information collected in the depths, indicating the sensitive, painful, or hyperalgesic (pain-sensitive) zones that are signs of a disorder that may be more or less serious and could be fairly new or chronic and longstanding. This round trip of information is known as *biological feedback.* It acts as a retroactive system that ensures that the whole body is monitored and regulated as needed. Thus a specific skin zone "metamerically" reflects its organ counterpart, i.e., specific skin zones mirror their organ counterpart.

The Reflexology Treatment

We know that the human hand, like the foot, is a microcosm of the human body in its entirety. This is true not only physically, but emotionally, mentally, and temporally as well. The hand bears the stigmata of a person's past and the promise of his or her future. This is something the therapist should keep in mind when working with a patient.

Before beginning any treatment, it is extremely important to examine the hand and evaluate its condition. This should be based on your own good sense and intuition. It is of course common sense to avoid practicing reflexology on someone suffering from a contagious disease, given the risk of transmitting that illness to you. As well, caution is called for when treating people with degenerative diseases or grave physical disorders that are immunosuppressive: cancer, AIDS, serious bronchial blockages, and anything that contributes to the deterioration of the body, including internal and cerebral hemorrhages. However, it is possible to provide relief for pain, stress, and fear. The method of total reflexology therapy outlined in this book allows people to better tolerate their functional disorders and the pain caused by illnesses of physiological origin and by the medications used to treat those serious illnesses.

In providing treatment, the therapist must be particularly attentive to the following:

▶ In treating people with rheumatoid polyarthritis and other forms of arthritis caused by the inflammation of the intra-articular spaces, manipulations can pose a risk of being painful and causing injury. Be sensitive and use caution in treating, all the while monitoring the person's response.

▶ When cuts, sprains, blisters, scabs, skin outbreaks, whitlow, any kind of infection, or cracked skin is present, the area of concern should be meticulously examined according to its location in the zone to be treated, and worked on without applying too much pressure.

▶ When treating swollen areas that are painful to the touch, work above or below or around the area in question.

▶ In the case of frostbite, Raynaud's disease, or simply when the person has extremely cold hands, devote more time to preparation as well as to performing manipulations used for warming and for concluding a session. Equal care should be given to the fragile hands of the very old and the very young.

▶ In the case of nervous-system diseases, especially Parkinson's and the delirium tremens caused by the abuse of alcohol, use a firm grip but apply a light, delicate pressure.

▶ Strict boundaries must be established when treating any person affected by a mental disorder.

▶ The reflexologist should guard against talking too much during a treatment and should not seek to intervene, interfere, or otherwise impose him- or herself on the client.

► At all times constantly bear in mind that you are treating a person, not a disease.

Initial Observations of the Patient

Take note of the person's history, including illnesses and surgeries and all past and present treatments. Then feel his or her occipital zones, studying his or her morphotype (somatotypes such as ectomorphic, endomorphic, and mesomorphic) as well as analyzing the person's level of stress. Subsequently the therapist should consider the various treatment options according to the pathologies of the systems involved. It is important to distinguish

► the symptom, whether perceived by the client/patient or established by another clinical practitioner

► the syndrome (the group of symptoms) that indicates the pathological process

► the illness (the combination of syndromes)

Be sure to review, from both an anatomical as well as a general health perspective, the principles of the skeletal, digestive, urinary, respiratory, cardiovascular, and lymphatic systems when making your initial observations. Attention should be given to Hering's law when monitoring the progression of a treatment: recall that the symptoms should move from top to bottom (descend); from inside to outside (exit); and from present toward the past (reliving earlier experiences).

The Clinical Appearance of the Hand

Observe the form and color of the hand and take note of any imperfections, including the following:

► calluses, warts, scars, damaged nails (if warts are present, note whether viral in origin, indicating a deficiency)

► fungal infections (indicating an imbalance of the pH of secretions)

► hyperkeratosis (a thickening of the outer layer of the skin, which indicates a need to eliminate toxins, which are best done prior to reflexology treatment)

► damp skin (indicating strong emotions or an autonomic nerve disorder)

► skin temperature (indicating the state of the circulation)

Be a Good Listener

Above all, the therapist must know how to listen; this is of critical importance. This listening must be active and deeply attentive. Listening to the person without judging or interrupting or changing the subject is the key to good listening. Any answers to the patient's questions should be spontaneous (as opposed to previously thought out or scripted) and spoken in a calm cadence. Do not try to rush the person as he or she talks, as trust is important in any healing process.

The Treatment

Once the patient is comfortably seated or lying down, you can begin the session.

To start out, a short hand-warming massage will help the person relax while preparing his or her hand for stimulating the reflex points. Place the hand to be given treatment in the desired position. Take off your watch and any jewelry and ask your patient to do the same. The best way to proceed is to place the person's palm or the dorsal surface of the hand on top of a cushion, although this is not absolutely necessary provided you and the person are both comfortable.

Hold the person's right hand in both of your hands, with your thumbs parallel and against each other on the back (dorsal side) of the person's hand, right in the center. Slide your thumbs toward the sides of the hand while gently opening toward the metacarpal bones. Gently pull on each finger and thumb, then rotate them once before placing them back on the cushion. Take the person's hand between your hands and turn it over, palm upward.

Now place your thumb on the solar plexus reflex point that is located almost dead center in the palm and exert a gentle but sustained pressure. Repeat this on the other hand.

Pick up the right hand again, palm down, facing the cushion. Fold your fingers under, and with your thumb beneath the person's hand, massage the wrist. Cup the joints on the back of the person's hand with your own hand.

Make a fist with your hand and place it beneath the palm. Knead the palm with your fist making a short circular movement. This massage helps relax the joints and makes them more flexible so they can be worked on. Repeat this movement on the left hand and turn over both hands.

Place your fingertips on those of the patient and repeat the movement that you made during the initial warming massage, but with both your hands this time. Go up the arm and back down toward the hand while pulling the thumbs toward the bottom. Repeat this three times. While you perform this technique, listen carefully to the quality of the movement of the cerebrospinal fluid at the cranial level (see page 51). After determining which zones to treat, the reflex treatment is performed by pressing your thumb on the zone to be treated, moving it in a circular motion, without removing it from the skin. This pattern mimics the helicoidal movement of the DNA.

Give yourself twenty to thirty minutes to effectively perform a full session on each hand. A reflexology treatment on both hands will therefore last one hour.

How Much Pressure Should Be Exerted?

On a scale from 1 to 3, the pressure you exert should go from light to strong. Pressing more intensely works better on the palms than on the backs of the hands, because the dorsal side contains many blood vessels, ligaments, and tendons and can be hurt if manipulated too forcefully. Determine what the person's particular pain threshold is and remain below that. For this reason it is vital to establish a relationship of trust with your patient. Observe the person's face as you work. It is essential to take it easy when working on sensitive regions, manipulating them slowly at first, and stretching the skin, as the reflex points are often deeply buried. Only then should pressure be increased, but not enough to go beyond the person's tolerance.

In some cases, manipulations will have to be adapted in accordance with the patient's age or state of health, as follows:

Young children: Exert only a very light pressure and keep the session short. It's best that an adult (mother or father, or another close relative) is present. Offer the child a toy while getting the history from the parents, so as to provide a relaxed environment for the child in which a playful rather than a solemn approach prevails. There should be no hesitation about pursuing this approach in establishing trust with a young person.

The elderly or those with delicate health: Employ lighter than usual pressure. Adopt a slower rhythm, and do not apply any force to specific reflex points. More time should be devoted to relaxation techniques and less to manipulations, and take time to put the person at ease.

Terminal patients: For those who have been diagnosed with a terminal illness, use light pressure aimed at soothing pain. The session should be short but treatments should be given more frequently, and greater time should be spent comforting and relaxing the person.

Nervous and anxious patients: For anyone exhibiting signs of nervousness or anxiety, provide reassurance about the painless nature of the hand reflexology treatment and describe its many benefits, particularly the relaxation effect.

Carpal tunnel syndrome: This common disorder should not be considered a counterindication for a hand reflexology session, but it does mean that a lighter treatment should be given to the back of the hand and no treatment whatsoever given to the zones of the wrist located above the palmar bones.

Ending the Session

Once the session has ended, listen again to the cerebrospinal fluid. Ask the person to take several deep, conscious breaths and to take a few moments to enter into a state of deep relaxation.

The session should last around an hour (unless otherwise indicated). At the end of the session, the first reaction that you will likely observe in the person is that she or he will seem to feel cold. Shivering, yawning, and stretching are frequent reactions. The more enduring effects, over a longer period of time, will involve liver, gallbladder, kidneys, and skin detoxification. The person will recover at his or her own pace, based on a capacity for openness and receptivity as well as the chronic nature of his or her condition.

Be aware that some medications can alter the body's reaction to reflexology treatments.

Afterward

In the beginning, the body can react with a strong but passing aggravation of symptoms or with the appearance of new, acute ones. This is what is known as a *healing crisis* (and the patient should be advised that this is a positive sign). In the normal order of things this is almost always followed by an improvement in the person's health. This should be considered a decisive moment in the treatment course.

Furthermore, it has been observed by veteran reflexologists that depending on the illness or disorder, reflex work on the hands generally proves to be even more effective than foot reflexology. This is particularly true for all physical syndromes that manifest above the waist, while the feet remain the preferred zone for treatment of syndromes affecting the body below the waist.

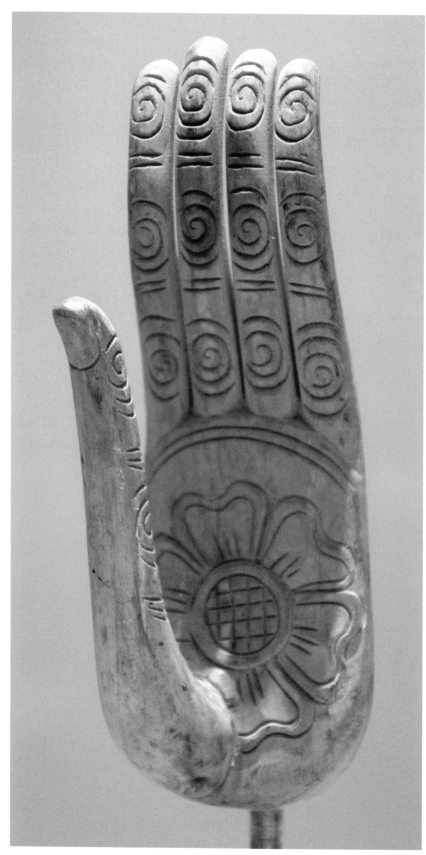

Wooden sculpture from Indonesia—anterior face of hand

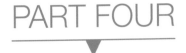

PART FOUR

Hand Reflexology

And the Systems
and Energy Centers of the Body

If cattle and horses, or lions, had hands, or were able to draw
with their feet and produce the works which men do,
horses would draw the forms of gods like horses, and cattle like cattle,
and they would make the gods' bodies the same shape as their own.

XENOPHANES

The Craniosacral System

Neural oscillations, the rhythmic or repetitive neural activity in the central nervous system, create a network of correlations. These complex waves are picked up by the cells, broken down into simple waves, and translated into electrical impulses or frequencies. The brain vibrates on scales of various frequencies, which may be harmonious or not. The pineal gland is the central point, the transmitter and receiver of vibrations. Bones, membranes, and fluids play the role of sound box and selective amplifiers. The quality of this music depends on numerous factors:

► the quality of the sensory organs (transmitters)
► the state of the neurons and brain (the wealth of intra- and interhemispherical connections)
► cellular reverberation and marking (acquired or transmitted memory, selections and knowledge learned earlier)
► the resonant qualities of the skull, whose shape, plasticity, and density modify the fringes of the correlations
► holographic reconstructions from simple waves
► the quality of captured frequencies (range, coherency, intensity)
► the motivation and attention of the subject, the major functions of consciousness

This information is shared as vibrations by all parts of the brain and therefore in all parts of the body.

The thumbs reflect the entire brain, with the right hemisphere on the right thumb and the left hemisphere on the left. This "brain map" found on the hands includes the neocortex, the limbic system, the reptilian brain, the hippocampus, the amygdala nuclei, the emotional relays, and the mammillary tubercules. Reflexology has access to each structure and system. By working on the brain membranes (the dura mater, the arachnoid, and the pia mater), the falx of the cerebrum, and the tentorium of the cerebellum, one can bring improvement to memory problems, phobias, and so on.

The brain is also mirrored on the other fingers of both hands. It is on these fingers that the reflexologist should work to treat the sutures, membranes, and cranial nerves. It has even been noted, for example, that in cases of a cerebral vascular stroke it is possible to detect the original zones of the hemorrhaged lesions on the fingers.

Working on the Craniosacral Rhythm

Working on the craniosacral rhythm means treating the effects caused by disruptive factors such as emotional, mental, or physical shocks; prolonged stress; and chronic, long-lasting illness. Before approaching the patient, the reflexologist should have in mind the integration and holistic nature of the primary respiratory mechanism that travels from the bones of the skull through the spinal column into the sacrum, before terminating at the hands and feet, integrating with all the tissues.

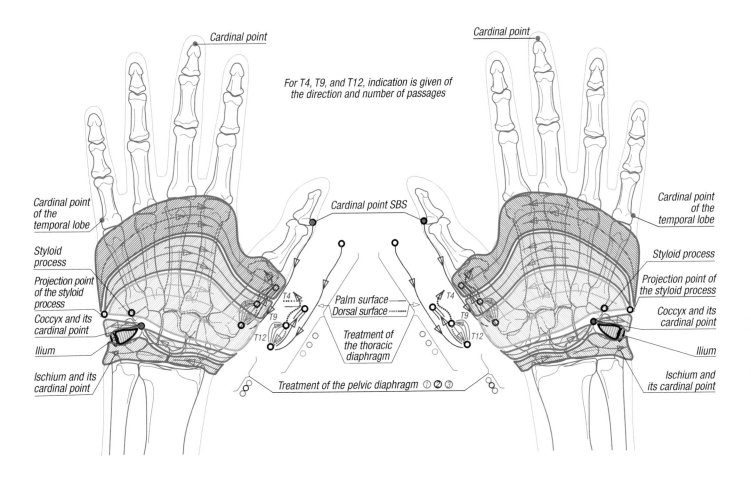

RIGHT PALM SURFACE

LEFT PALM SURFACE

Cardinal point

Cardinal point

For T4, T9, and T12, indication is given of the direction and number of passages

Cardinal point of the temporal lobe

Cardinal point SBS

Cardinal point of the temporal lobe

Styloid process

Styloid process

Projection point of the styloid process

Projection point of the styloid process

Coccyx and its cardinal point

Coccyx and its cardinal point

Ilium

Ilium

Ischium and its cardinal point

Ischium and its cardinal point

T4

T9

T12

T4

T9

T12

Palm surface ——
Dorsal surface ······

Treatment of the thoracic diaphragm

Treatment of the pelvic diaphragm ① ② ③

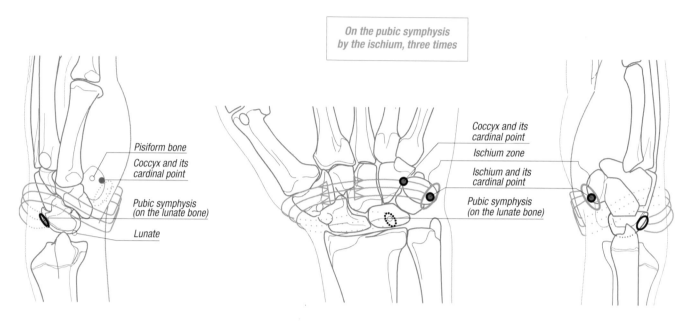

On the pubic symphysis
by the ischium, three times

Pisiform bone

Coccyx and its
cardinal point

Pubic symphysis
(on the lunate bone)

Lunate

Coccyx and its
cardinal point

Ischium zone

Ischium and its
cardinal point

Pubic symphysis
(on the lunate bone)

INNER LATERAL SURFACE　　　**LEFT PALM SURFACE (RIGHT IDEM)**　　　*OUTER LATERAL SURFACE*

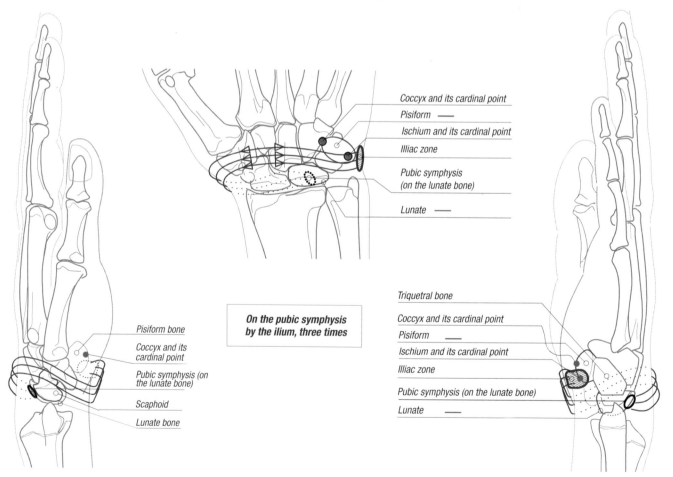

Coccyx and its cardinal point

Pisiform ——

Ischium and its cardinal point

Illiac zone

Pubic symphysis
(on the lunate bone)

Lunate ——

On the pubic symphysis
by the ilium, three times

Pisiform bone

Coccyx and its
cardinal point

Pubic symphysis (on
the lunate bone)

Scaphoid

Lunate bone

Triquetral bone

Coccyx and its cardinal point

Pisiform ——

Ischium and its cardinal point

Illiac zone

Pubic symphysis (on the lunate bone)

Lunate ——

At the initial consultation, the therapist will take the cranial pulse, listening to the quality of the cerebrospinal fluid and measuring the pulsations of the PRM. By feeling the client's hands, the therapist measures the symmetry, quality, rate, and amplitude of the fluid movement underneath the fingers. If the therapist's hands perceive a jerky and not fluid movement of the PRM or cerebrospinal fluid, it can be certain that the person is in a state of constant suffering. It is only when the fluid, smooth movement of the primary respiratory mechanism is restored and the entire body is irrigated that the reflexology treatment has done its job.

The following points of the skull can be located on the hand:

▶ the junction of the temporal, parietal, and occipital bones; the sphenoid and ethmoid bones
▶ the junction of the coronal and sagittal sutures
▶ the external occipital protuberance
▶ the junction of the occipital, parietal, and sagittal sutures
▶ the junction of the frontal, parietal, sphenoid, and temporal bones

Work on all these areas is a must.

Working on the Connective Tissue

Reflexology assists the vital force in the restoration of the connective tissue by relaxing the contracted muscle, normalizing fibrous tension, facilitating the elimination of scarring, and restoring the elasticity of stretched tissues. It therefore encourages the return of circulation to all parts of the body, drains stasis from a variety of areas, relaxes the vaso-sympathetic spasm, and regulates the nerve flow intended for the muscles and viscera.

Recent findings on the structural zones of the hands and feet have considerably expanded the therapeutic tool kit reflexology now offers for the treatment of autonomic nervous system disorders. Through craniosacral techniques and the stimulation of cerebrospinal fluid, reflexology restores homeostasis in the fasciae in cases of whiplash, which are responsible for highly painful zones in the connective tissue. What we witness as a result is

▶ a pumping of venous blood by the aponeurotic fascia
▶ a draining of serous fluids by evacuation through the lymphatic system
▶ a pumping of intra-bone fluids
▶ a wringing out of the sinus veins of parenchymatous fluids and cerebrospinal fluid by the fasciae and dura mater

When someone experiences an emotional shock, the body is effected by tension in its tissues that imprints itself on the fasciae. According to John Upledger (1932–2012), who developed craniosacral therapy in the 1970s as an offshoot of osteopathy, trauma is registered in the connective tissue as aqueous or energy cysts that remain throughout a person's lifetime or until removed by therapy. The emotional memory is charged by all the suffering the person has experienced. This suffering forms the foundation of experience and penetrates the unconscious. It can be removed, however, by a variety of methods, thus reestablishing emotional freedom. Like craniosacral therapy, reflexology, through the massage of the palms and soles, can erase the tensions and lead to a resurgence of an emotional memory.

Hering's law says that the deepest layers of the fasciae record memories going back to infancy, while the more superficial layers hold memories of more recent experiences. Over the course of a series of reflexology treatments, the person will often relive—through symptoms that reemerge in an incomprehensible guise—dreams, forgotten sensations, pains, irritants, and poorly handled experiences that have been recorded unconsciously but never expressed. Releasing these repressed experiences results in a feeling of liberation, both physical and emotional, if not true healing.

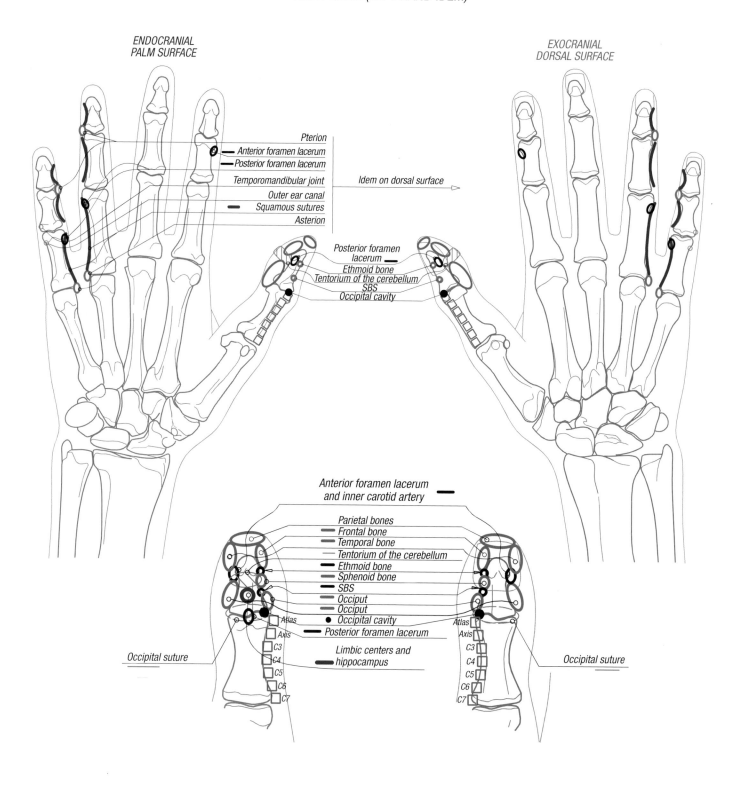

RIGHT HAND (LEFT HAND IDEM)

ENDOCRANIAL
PALM SURFACE

EXOCRANIAL
DORSAL SURFACE

Pterion
Anterior foramen lacerum
Posterior foramen lacerum
Temporomandibular joint
Outer ear canal
Squamous sutures
Asterion

Idem on dorsal surface →

Posterior foramen
lacerum
Ethmoid bone
Tentorium of the cerebellum
SBS
Occipital cavity

Anterior foramen lacerum
and inner carotid artery

Parietal bones
Frontal bone
Temporal bone
Tentorium of the cerebellum
Ethmoid bone
Sphenoid bone
SBS
Occiput
Occiput
Occipital cavity
Posterior foramen lacerum

Atlas
Axis
C3
C4
C5
C6
C7

Atlas
Axis
C3
C4
C5
C6
C7

Occipital suture

Occipital suture

Limbic centers and
hippocampus

RIGHT HAND (LEFT HAND IDEM)

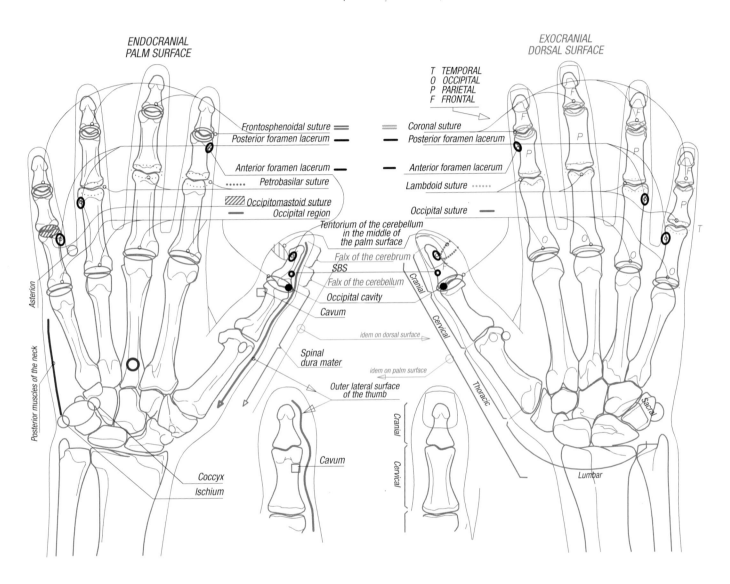

ENDOCRANIAL
PALM SURFACE

EXOCRANIAL
DORSAL SURFACE

T TEMPORAL
O OCCIPITAL
P PARIETAL
F FRONTAL

Frontosphenoidal suture ══
Posterior foramen lacerum ━

══ Coronal suture
Posterior foramen lacerum ━

Anterior foramen lacerum ━
Petrobasilar suture ‥‥‥

━ Anterior foramen lacerum
Lambdoid suture ‥‥‥

▨ Occipitomastoid suture
━ Occipital region

Occipital suture ━

Tentorium of the cerebellum
in the middle of
the palm surface
Falx of the cerebrum
SBS
Falx of the cerebellum
Occipital cavity
Cavum

Cranial
Cervical
Thoracic

idem on dorsal surface

Spinal
dura mater

idem on palm surface

Outer lateral surface
of the thumb

Asterion

Posterior muscles of the neck

Cavum

Cranial
Cervical

Coccyx
Ischium

Cavum

Sacral

Lumbar

Finally, massage of the sphenobasilar point on the hand activates and regulates cranial articulations and cerebrospinal fluid. This is how it balances the sacrum and skull connected by the core link, or spinal column, and the cerebrospinal fluid.

Here, the operating principle of this therapy is the transfer of the therapist's electrical nature into the patient. This phenomenon can be observed in all the natural therapies that involve vital energy, prana, or *chi* of traditional Chinese medicine, including reflexology. What we find here is the mind-body duality resolving into oneness. The reflexologist works the vital energies with flexibility and an open mind in order to observe the new facts that emerge under his or her fingers.

Resolving the Pain of Stress

Stress is defined as "a constraining force or influence," "physical force or pressure," and "something that causes strong feelings of worry and anxiety." Stress is the body's natural response to a stressor. It is born from the shock caused by the collision of two opposing forces that are unable to merge, hence the tension produced by stress.

Stress characterizes almost every aspect of our lives. It can engender psychological disorders like anxiety and depression, as well as psychosomatic pathologies. Many forms of imbalance can be directly tied to it and are aggravated by its effects. If it cannot be dealt with adequately when it first appears, despite the unpleasantness it creates, there is a risk it will lead to harsh physical afflictions. If stress is prolonged and chronic, the body rebuilds its nutritional reserves more slowly, which makes it more vulnerable to attack, thereby delaying healing. Combatting the effects of stress is one of the major objectives of reflexology, which explains why it contributes so greatly to creating a state of overall relaxation that is propitious for recovery.

To clearly understand how reflexology works to reduce the effects of stress, we must first understand the dynamics of pain. The skin and blood vessels contain thousands of nerve endings that react to various kinds of stimuli such as cuts, stings, heat, burns, stretching, or pressure. The pain receptors scatter throughout the body to spread the warning of a possible wound. Fear and anxiety are emotional states that are also associated with pain and pain thresholds, which can vary wildly from one person to the next.

Referred pain is the name given to pain that is projected beyond the site of the initial injury or pathological zone. It is produced because the sensitive nerves converge before entering the brain, causing confusion as to the exact source of the pain. For example, dental pain is perceived in the ear because they share a common innervation; a vesicular pain is felt for the same reason in the area of the shoulder blade. Stress in many ways exhibits all the signs of referred pain, by expressing itself in disease and other forms of imbalance.

A person's state of mind is closely linked to his or her physical well-being. Negative emotional states such as those caused by stress will find expression in pain and physical disorders if we do not address the root cause. Practicing deep breathing and quieting the mind is, of course, essential to calming the emotions. Reflexology is also an invaluable tool for finding relief from the pain of stress.

To address all matters relating to stress, stimulate the reflex points corresponding to the following anatomical zones:

▶ cranial nerves
▶ diaphragm
▶ neck
▶ pineal gland
▶ hypothalamus
▶ spinal column
▶ lungs
▶ large intestine
▶ kidneys and adrenals

Craniosacral Reflexology

Emotional Organic Zones of the Center of the Hand

PALM AND LATERAL SURFACES

LEFT PALM SURFACE (RIGHT IDEM)

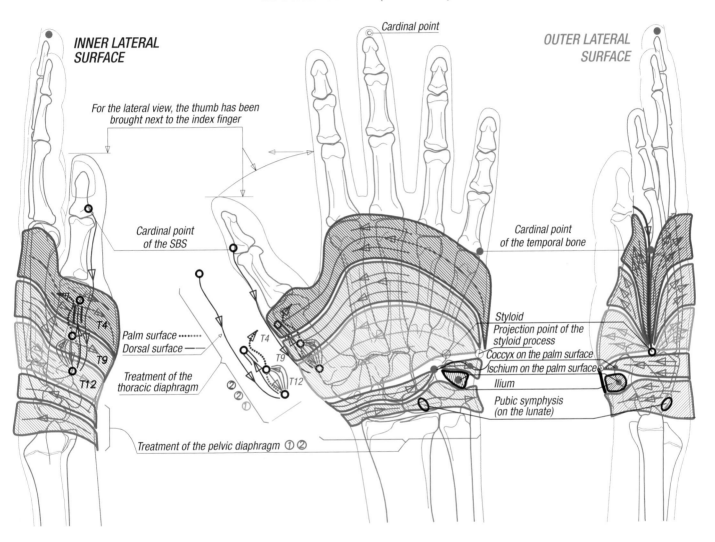

INNER LATERAL SURFACE

Cardinal point

OUTER LATERAL SURFACE

For the lateral view, the thumb has been brought next to the index finger

Cardinal point of the SBS

Cardinal point of the temporal bone

Palm surface ········
Dorsal surface ——

T4

T9

T12

Styloid
Projection point of the styloid process
Coccyx on the palm surface
Ischium on the palm surface
Ilium

Treatment of the thoracic diaphragm

Pubic symphysis (on the lunate)

Treatment of the pelvic diaphragm ① ②

For T4, T9, and T12, indication is given of the direction and number of passages

DORSAL AND LATERAL SURFACES

LEFT DORSAL SURFACE (RIGHT IDEM)

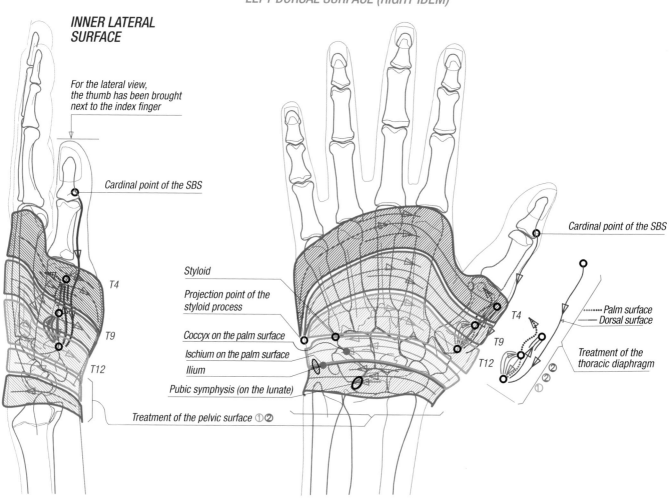

INNER LATERAL SURFACE

For the lateral view, the thumb has been brought next to the index finger

Cardinal point of the SBS

T4

T9

T12

Cardinal point of the SBS

Styloid

Projection point of the styloid process

Coccyx on the palm surface

Ischium on the palm surface

Ilium

Pubic symphysis (on the lunate)

Treatment of the pelvic surface ①②

T4

T9

T12

Palm surface
Dorsal surface

Treatment of the thoracic diaphragm

①②
①

For T4, T9, and T12, indication is given of the direction and number of passages

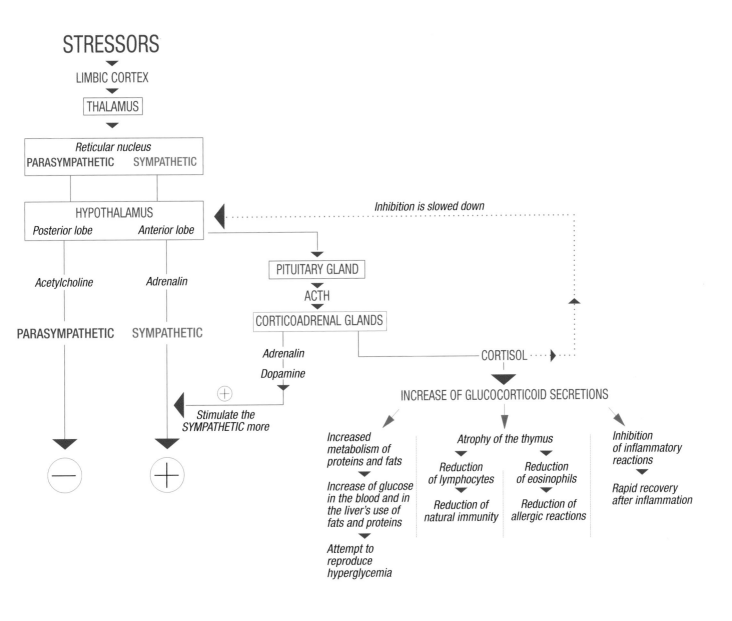

Again, always remember Hering's law in practicing reflexology: Everything that is below exists above. Symptoms evolve from the outside toward the inside when an illness becomes more aggravated, and from the inside outward when the situation improves. The aggravated state is characterized by an upward movement from bottom to top, and improvement is signaled by movement in the reverse direction from the top to the bottom. Above all, remember that the resurgence of symptoms from a past illness or disorder is actually a herald of improved health.

Whiplash

A considerable number of problems can appear following whiplash, which covers not only the notion of the "rabbit punch" associated with a sudden sharp whipping movement of the neck and head (as of a person in a vehicle that is struck head-on or from the rear by another vehicle), but also all the psychic, mental, and emotional trauma that goes with it that affects the whole of the human body. Often ignored because the original incident seems insignificant at the time, whiplash can go unnoticed, and the person can undergo countless medical examinations that will produce no conclusive results.

The frequency of psychic, sensory, and motor disorders should all call attention to an original trauma of whiplash. The following regions are most frequently involved:

Parietal region: A trauma in this zone causes troubles with coordination and motor function (poor control of voluntary movements, loss of equilibrium, apraxia).

Frontal and prefrontal region: As the frontal and prefrontal areas are the centers for expression of consciousness, intelligence, and character, there might be radical changes in behavior in these areas. Trauma to this zone can also cause poor tactile recognition and troubles with perception.

Sphenoid region: An injury to the sphenoid bone, which protects the pituitary gland, can cause serious problems affecting growth, ossification, sexual disorders (dysmenorrhea), and metabolic, vagal (relating to the vagus nerve), and behavioral disorders. The relationship of the small wings with the Broca's area (a brain

Stress Syndrome on the Hands

FUNCTIONAL STEPS		ORGANIC STEPS	
ALARM	ADAPTATION	CHRONIC STATE	EXHAUSTION
Sympathetic	Sympathetic and parasympathetic system	Parasympathetic system ↗ for acute crisis	Sympathetic ↘ and parasympathetic ↘ systems
Pain +++ No contraction Tissues can be massaged more deeply	Generalized pain not fixed to any location +++ Tissue contraction Hardening of tissues Granulation	Localized fixed pain +++ Contractions = cords Points sink deeper Hypersecretion	Pain that is acute Floppy feet
Calm by working on the para-sympathetic system through: – Cranial zones – Pituitary gland – Solar plexus – Adrenal glands – Sacrum	To be worked first : – The dorsal column (sympathetic system) – Solar plexus – End with the parasympathetic system	Use general treatment for acute crisis Work on sympathetic system +++	Light general treatment on the sympathetic and parasym-pathetic systems

The Six Stages of Stress Syndrome

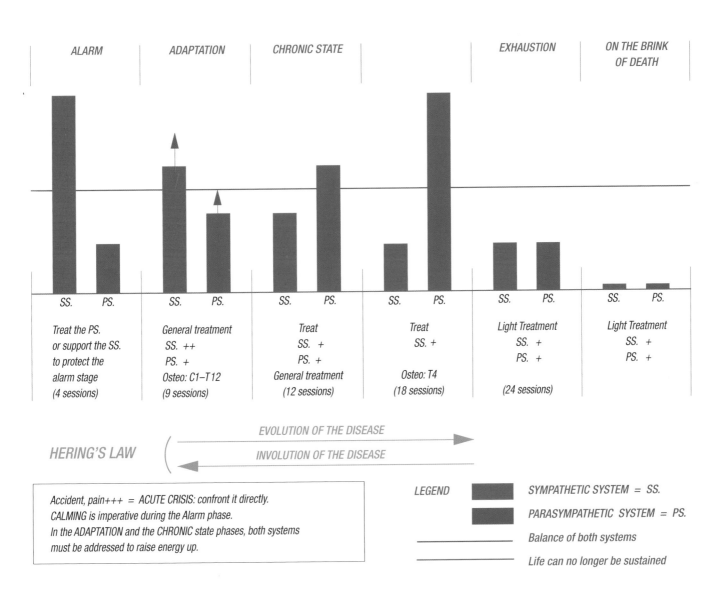

ALARM	ADAPTATION	CHRONIC STATE		EXHAUSTION	ON THE BRINK OF DEATH
SS. PS.	SS. PS.	SS. PS.	SS. PS.	SS. PS.	SS. PS.
Treat the PS. or support the SS. to protect the alarm stage (4 sessions)	General treatment SS. ++ PS. + Osteo: C1–T12 (9 sessions)	Treat SS. + PS. + General treatment (12 sessions)	Treat SS. + Osteo: T4 (18 sessions)	Light Treatment SS. + PS. + (24 sessions)	Light Treatment SS. + PS. +

HERING'S LAW

EVOLUTION OF THE DISEASE →

INVOLUTION OF THE DISEASE ←

Accident, pain+++ = ACUTE CRISIS: confront it directly.
CALMING is imperative during the Alarm phase.
In the ADAPTATION and the CHRONIC state phases, both systems
must be addressed to raise energy up.

LEGEND

SYMPATHETIC SYSTEM = SS.

PARASYMPATHETIC SYSTEM = PS.

Balance of both systems

Life can no longer be sustained

center associated with the motor control of speech and usually located in the left but sometimes in the right inferior frontal gyrus) will result in problems with language, while the greater wings that are connected with the taste centers can cause a disruption of these centers. An injury to the fulcrum between the occiput/sphenoid and the sphenobasilar symphysis can be the cause of migraines and headaches.

Temporal region: The temporal lobe contains the auditory-receptive area; trauma here can result in psychic hearing loss, ringing in the ears, Ménière's disease, facial neuralgia, and problems relating to symbolic thought and language.

Sphenobasilar region: The hypothalamus is located at the base of the brain, on the floor of the third ventricle. Through its nerve connection with the higher brain, it plays an important role in mental disorders and insomnia. Trauma in this region can result in the person exhibiting aggressive behavior alternating with fear and anger.

Occipital region: This area corresponds to the structural visual area and trauma there can cause hallucinations and distortions in spatial perception. The occipital cavity, through its membranous connections with the sacrum, sometimes causes nerve pain due to the compression of numerous nerve zones.

Orbital area: The cranial nerves III, IV, V, and VI pass through the sphenoidal fissure. Shrinkage of this area can cause congestion to the ocular globe with hypermetropia, myopia, astigmatism, and strabism.

The Three Diaphragms and Their Balance

There are three major diaphragms: the respiratory diaphragm, located at the base of the lungs, which aids in breathing; the pelvic diaphragm, located at the pelvic floor, which is important in elimination of solid and liquid waste; and the vocal diaphragm, located at the throat, which controls breathing and speaking.

Most of the areas that shape the course of the fasciae follow more of a longitudinal rather than a transverse direction. They are characterized by a very slight gliding mobility, a slight glide that is more visible in the longitudinal direction than the transverse one. The most visible of the structures of potential restriction is the respiratory diaphragm, which separates the thoracic cavity from the abdominal cavity. It is essentially a fibrous myoseptum. The central tendon is the link on the front of the body that connects the three diaphragms, a counterpart to the core link, or spinal column, on the back of the body. It is their combined action that allows a person to resist the effects of gravity.

When the respiratory diaphragm's muscle contracts, it pulls the semicircular band lower, thereby reducing intrathoracic pressure by increasing the volume. At the same time it increases the intra-abdominal pressure and reduces the volume. A contraction of the respiratory diaphragm exerts traction directed downward on the pericardium, a traction that is echoed via the continuity of the fascia on the base of the skull by the carotid sheath that surrounds the vascular compartment of the neck.

The diaphragm is innervated by the branches of the primary ventral divisions of the ninth through twelfth spinal dorsal nerves, and by the phrenic nerve, which emerges from the fourth cervical nerve but is also capable of sharing anastomoses with the third and fifth spinal cervical nerves. The hypertonia, or contraction, of the respiratory diaphragm can be unilateral or bilateral, resulting from problems associated with one of the four spinal dorsal nerves, with a loss of mobility in the fascia. This will lead to a loss of vitality in the patient, which will be the source of all kinds of weaknesses, ill-defined states of fatigue, and migraines, which cause the toxic wastes due to the lessened mobility of fluidic and gaseous exchanges to accumulate, which in turn causes depression and a general state of malaise. Poor mobility of the craniosacral system can also be noted among patients displaying chronic tension (hypertonicity) of the diaphragm.

To reduce this tension and reduce this pressure to move lower, thereby freeing the primary respiratory mechanism, the central tendon should be treated. It can be worked on in zone 1 at the level of T4, T5, T6, on the reflex zone of the xiphoid process.

The Three Levels of Being and Their Treatment in Reflexology

Reflexology has the effect of reducing deep blockages that have the potential to become the source of future disorders. The results of reflexology treatments can be evaluated in accordance with the criteria established by Hering's law: from the top to the bottom; from the inside to the outside; from the present to the past.

Reflexology treatment of the craniosacral system should only be undertaken after the practitioner has obtained a holistic understanding of the patient with the help of general protocols that permit the reflexologist to regulate the different systems involved. As a priority the practitioner should treat the membranes (dura mater, arachnoid, pia mater), the cranial sutures, the cranial nerves, the three diaphragms, the plexuses, and depending on the patient, the therapy should end with treatment of the cerebral or pelvic zones.

The Physical Level, or Tentorium Sacrum

The tentorium sacrum is one of three tentorium (the other two being the tentorium cerebellum and the tentorium medium); it is located on the pisiform bone and mirrors the structure of the cells, nerves, chemical mediators, fluids, tissues, fasciae, and organs. The tentorium sacrum contains two plexuses:

► the coccygeal plexus connected with sexuality and reproduction

► the hypogastric plexus connected to the adrenal glands

Treatment of the tentorium sacrum is performed on the reflex zones of the coccyx, the pubic rim, the iliopubic ramus, the ischiopubic ramus, the obturator foramen, and the sciatic spine.

We will now examine all the minor diaphragms of the pelvis in order to treat the tentorium sacrum. The pelvic diaphragm is made up of muscles that lift the anus, coccygeal muscles, and their fasciae. It extends like a hammock through the pelvis, where it serves as a support to the pelvic viscera. The anus, ureter, and vagina cross through it.

The urogenital diaphragm consists of the fasciae of several muscles that cross through the pelvis.

The coccygeal muscle is formed from sinewy muscle fibers. It originates in the sciatic spine and the large sacrosciatic ligament. It fits through the sacral-coccygeal joint. It is innervated by the branches of the plexus pudendus coming out of the fourth and fifth sacral segments. The coccygeal muscle pulls on the coccyx and the sacral apex before this, thereby producing a flexion within the craniosacral system.

The superficial leaf of the urogenital diaphragm is attached laterally to the branches of the pubis, on the arched subpubic ligaments, and on the ischiatic tuberosities. It also permits the passage of the ureter and vagina and forms part of their walls.

The muscles that fit in over the sacrum and which, through abnormal tension, can bring about a disruption of the craniosacral system, are primarily:

The iliac: The iliac muscle bends the thigh.

The gluteus maximus: A hypertonia of the gluteus maximus will create a loss of mobility in the sacrum.

The psoas-iliac: Successful decompression of the lumbosacral joint of the occipital-atlas region, as well as that of the sphenobasilar joint, routinely produces remarkable if not spectacular changes.

The Psychic Level (Emotional), or Tentorium Medium

This zone is found on the hand between C7/T1 to T12, the reflex headquarters for many organs: the

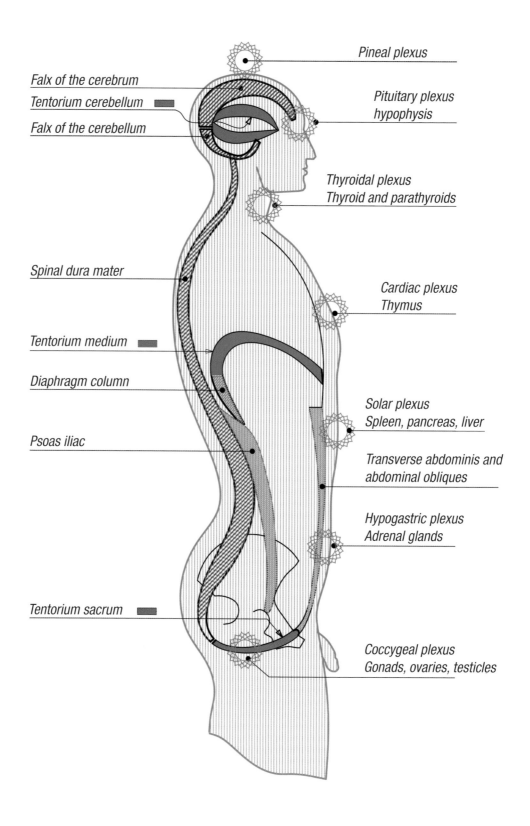

Pineal plexus

Falx of the cerebrum

Tentorium cerebellum ▬

Falx of the cerebellum

Pituitary plexus
hypophysis

Thyroidal plexus
Thyroid and parathyroids

Spinal dura mater

Cardiac plexus
Thymus

Tentorium medium ▬

Diaphragm column

Solar plexus
Spleen, pancreas, liver

Psoas iliac

Transverse abdominis and
abdominal obliques

Hypogastric plexus
Adrenal glands

Tentorium sacrum ▬

Coccygeal plexus
Gonads, ovaries, testicles

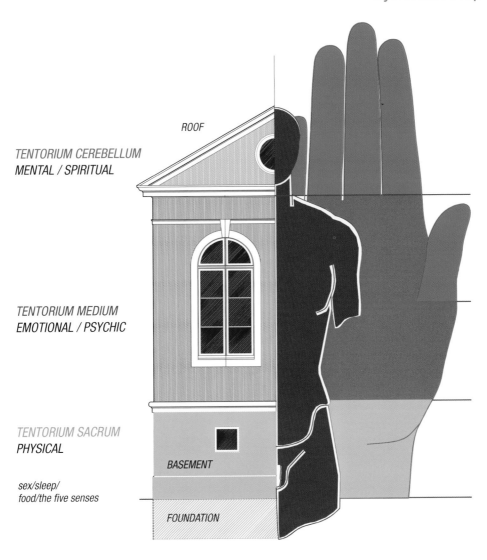

ROOF

TENTORIUM CEREBELLUM
MENTAL / SPIRITUAL

TENTORIUM MEDIUM
EMOTIONAL / PSYCHIC

TENTORIUM SACRUM
PHYSICAL

*sex/sleep/
food/the five senses*

BASEMENT

FOUNDATION

liver, stomach, spleen, pancreas, heart, lungs, kidneys, and adrenal glands. It is the digestion center as well as serving as an emotional reserve. The tentorium medium contains three plexuses:

▶ the solar plexus connected with the pancreas or liver
▶ the cardiac plexus connected to the thymus
▶ the thyroidal plexus connected to the thyroid and parathyroid glands

Treatment of the tentorium medium is performed on the zones of the diaphragm columns, the intercostals, the diaphragmatic cupola, and most particularly, on those of the cardium, stomach, and heart.

The Mental Level (Spiritual), or Tentorium Cerebellum

This area is mirrored on the fingers as well as between C1 and C7. It contains the sensory organs of sight, hearing, smell, and taste, which partially permit

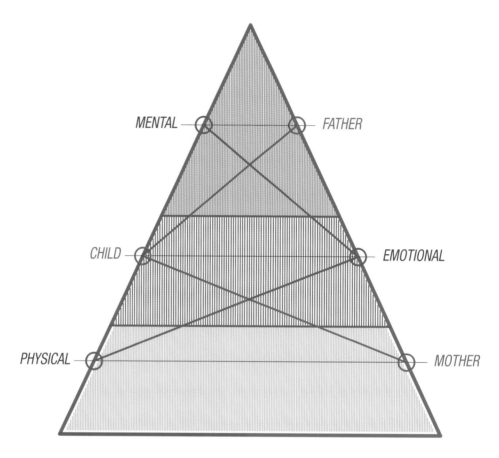

perception of the outside world from which the brain can get an idea of its surroundings. The degrees of perception and interpretation vary from one person to the next. The same holds true therefore for behaviors when confronting a fairly similar event. In some therapies treatment of this level is considered a priority. The tentorium cerebellum contains two plexuses:

▶ the cerebral plexus, whose corresponding gland is the pituitary

▶ the coronal plexus, which corresponds to the pineal gland

Treatment of the tentorium cerebellum is performed on the reflexology zones associated with the sphenobasilar symphysis, the falx of the cerebrum, the tentorium of the cerebellum, the rim of the occipital cavity, and the posterior foramen lacerum, as well as on the zones of the occipital, lambdoid, frontosphenoidal, petrobasilar, occipitomastoid, temporomandibular, and the parietal squamous sutures.

The Neuroendocrine System

For everything to function together, a global communication system that travels in both directions is necessary. This is the purpose of the neuroendocrine system, the interconnected nervous and endocrine systems. These two systems act together to regulate the physiological processes of the human body. Neuroendocrinology arose from the recognition that the brain, especially the hypothalamus, controls secretion of pituitary gland hormones. It has subsequently expanded to include the study of the numerous interconnections of the endocrine and nervous systems.

At the beginning of the twentieth century, English physiologist Ernest Starling (who among other contributions discovered peristalsis, introduced the concept of hormones, and described fluid shifts in the body) believed that the endocrine system and nervous system performed the same function: they assured communication between the different parts of the body and the outside, and coordinated the multiple functions necessary to life. The nervous system performed this function of integration quite rapidly. It sent messages to all parts of the body in the form of electrical signals that transited through the paths of the nerves. Starling maintained that the endocrine system did the same thing, but much more slowly because it used "chemical messengers" that traveled through the blood: hormones.

We know that the central organ for the nervous system is, of course, the brain. For the endocrine system, this central role was first assigned to the pituitary gland, then to the hypothalamus, then finally to the pineal gland.

The Endocrine Glands and Their Hormones

The endocrine system refers to the collection of glands that secrete chemical messengers called hormones directly into the circulatory system (the bloodstream) to be carried toward distant target organs (in contrast to the exocrine system, which secretes its hormones to the outside of the body using ducts). It was long thought that the nervous and endocrine systems worked independently. It was then discovered that two hypophyseal (relating to the pituitary gland) hormones, oxytocin and vasopressin, were synthesized in the hypothalamus before being transported by the nerve path into the pituitary gland. This organ simply stored and released them. This was how the concept of neurosecretion—the process of producing a secretion by nerve cells—was established.

The pituitary gland, a small spheroid-shaped organ, weighs about 0.5 grams in a human being. It is located in a bony cavity at the base of the skull, the sella turcica, where it is connected to the base of the skull by the pituitary stalk. The pituitary gland is formed by two lobes that are of different embryonic origin: the posterior lobe of the nerve origin (neurohypophyseal) and the anterior lobe. The first of these lobes releases the neurohormones oxytocin and vasopressin, which originate in two clumps of neurons that are neurosecretory, the supraoptic nucleus and paraventricular nucleus, located in the hypothalamus. Synthesized in the cellular bodies of these neurons, they are transported along the axons into the neurohypophysis (the neural lobe of the pituitary gland). There they are stored until they are released into the circulatory systems of the body as needed. Vasopressin is an antidiuretic hormone. It is employed for the reabsorption of water by the kidney tubules; it thereby allows water to be conserved and reduces urine volume. Damage to the neurohypophysis (by a tumor, for example) causes diabetes insipidus, which results in a substantial increase in thirst and urine volume. The hormone oxytocin causes the contraction of the smooth muscle fibers of the uterus during the birth process as well as that of the contractile tissues of the mammary gland during breastfeeding.

The anterior lobe of the pituitary gland, meanwhile, releases the hormones that control the peripheral endocrine glands. Thyrotropic hormone (TSH) controls the thyroid, gonadotropic hormones (luteinizing or LH and follicle-stimulating hormones, or FSH) control the gonads (ovaries and testicles), and the adrenocorticotropic hormone (ACTH) controls the cortico-adrenals. Human growth hormone (HGH) controls, as indicated by its name, growth. It does this in combination with other hormones or chemical factors (such as the growth factors called IGF, which are synthesized in large part by the liver, as well as by other tissues). Finally, prolactin plays an important role in the reproductive health of both men and women, as well as in lactation. It should be noted that no pituitary hormone controls the pancreas, which mainly releases insulin as well as other hormones.

Every thought and emotion affects our hormonal glands; if a disruption of any one of these seven glands occurs, the entire group suffers. Therefore, if we really want to realize our full potential as human beings, we should try to cultivate emotional equilibrium. Worries, fears, anxieties, resentments, and grief should give way to hope, courage, and joy, as one's state of mind has a positive effect on the optimal functioning of the hormonal glands.

The Pineal Gland

This gland is shaped like a cone and weighs around half an ounce. It is immersed in cerebrospinal fluid. Located behind the limbic brain, the pineal gland takes in the messages coming from other parts of the body. It releases melatonin, which, in addition to being linked to circadian rhythms, stimulates all other hormones and helps the glands respond to their messages.

The Hypothalamus

The hypothalamus forms the bridge between the pineal plexus and the pituitary plexus. It analyzes, balances, and transforms energy. It regulates growth thanks to GnRH, gonadotropin-releasing hormone. The hypothalamus plays a key role in the onset of sleep by two simultaneous operations: the activation of its anterior portion, the preoptic area, and the inhibition of the posterior hypothalamus involved in maintaining wakefulness. The dorsal raphe (on the midline of the brainstem) plays a role in the onset of sleep by releasing serotonin.

The Pituitary Gland

This gland is the size of a pea and weighs around 0.6 grams. It transmits hormonal stimulations to the other glands. The sella turcica, which holds the pituitary gland in the sphenoid bone, is stimulated by some target cells of the hypothalamus that were initially stimulated by the pineal gland. Nervous, hormonal, and emotional cycles are formed and organized by means of combined reactions. The pituitary gland releases four hormones: ACTH, GH, Prolactin, and TSH.

ACTH

ACTH, adrenocorticotropic hormone, is the stress hormone, produced in response to biological stress.

RIGHT PALM SURFACE

Pineal gland

Breasts
on the dorsal surface
Diaphragm
Liver
Gallbladder

Adrenals
Kidneys

Ovaries

Testicles

Hippocampus
Pituitary gland

Pineal gland
Hypothalamus
Parotid gland
Tonsils and adenoids
Parathyroids ●

Thyroid
Thymus

Pancreas

LEFT PALM SURFACE

Pineal gland

Pineal gland

Hypothalamus
Parotid gland
Tonsils and adenoids
Parathyroids ●

Hippocampus
Pituitary gland

Breasts
(on the dorsal surface)
Diaphragm
Liver

Spleen
Pancreas
Adrenals
Kidneys

Ovaries

Testicles

Thyroid
Thymus

Pancreas

Endocrine Glands and the Spinal Column

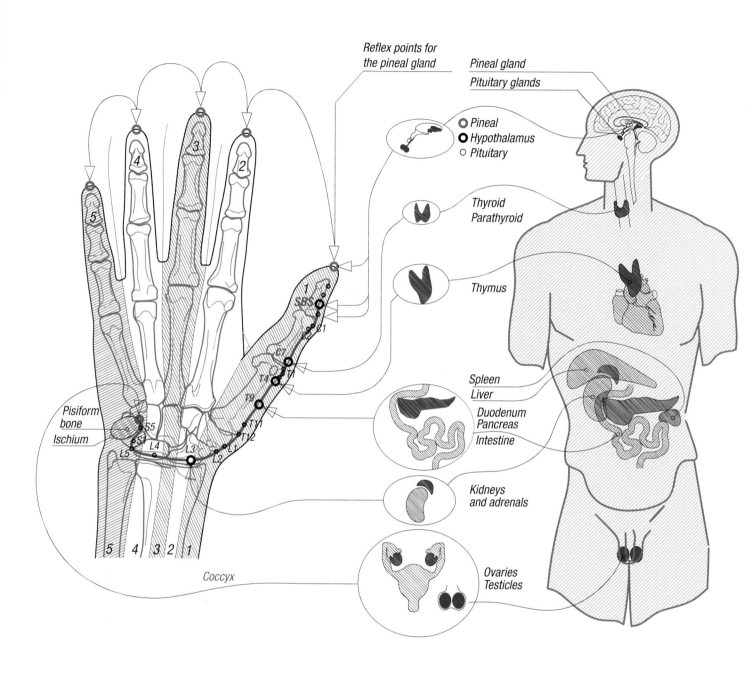

ACTH prompts the corticoadrenal glands to release glucocorticoids, the main one of which is cortisol. Along with adrenaline, it stimulates the breakdown of the glycogens stored in the liver and muscles into glucose, and that of the triglycerides in adipose tissue into glycerol and fatty acids. Once these elements have been broken down, they travel into the blood, forming an energy source the tissues can utilize. Cortisol also triggers the breakdown of proteins, releasing the amino acids used in the repair of injuries.

Growth Hormone

Also known as human growth hormone (HGH or hGH), this hormone completes the repairing activity of cortisol. Growth hormone is a protein consisting of ninety amino acids; 75 percent of the amount released in a twenty-four-hour period is done so at night, during slow, deep sleep. It is released by the pituitary gland under the principal influence of a hormone of the hypothalamus, GHRH (growth hormone releasing hormone). It is inhibited by another proteinic hormone, somatostatin. Growth hormone acts directly on the cells but also uses chemical intermediaries. The most important of these is IGF-1 (insulinlike growth factor 1).

After the first two decades of life, the GH level declines by an average of 14 percent every ten years because of the reduction of GHRH and other substances that stimulate growth hormone, because of the loss of sensitivity in the pituitary gland, and because of the increase of somatostatin. With the reduction of GH, the waistline grows larger and muscles atrophy. GH levels can also be reduced by

- ▶ obesity
- ▶ elevated blood sugar
- ▶ insufficient or restless sleep
- ▶ sleep apnea
- ▶ excessive consumption of aspirin
- ▶ estrogen taken orally

Prolactin

Also known as luteotropic hormone, or luteotropin, prolactin is a hypophyseal hormone. Its release increases toward the end of pregnancy, stimulating the production of milk by the mammary glands. It also plays a role in cellular division, reproduction, immunotherapy, and sexual behavior. Prolactin is important in the reproductive health of men too, however the specific function of this hormone in men is not well known (although levels of prolactin have been found to be a measure of sexual satisfaction in both men and women).

Thyroid-Stimulating Hormone (TSH)

Released by the pituitary gland in response to a stimulation of the hypothalamus, TSH plays a role in the regulation of body temperature. Its release is complex as it is connected to both circadian cycles and to sleep. Its production rate falls during deep sleep. Through the thyroid, it triggers the release of hormones that increase the production of heat through oxidation of nutrients in the cells.

The Thyroid and the Parathyroids

The thyroid is one of the largest endocrine glands in the body. It consists of two connected lobes found in the neck, below the laryngeal prominence (Adam's apple). The thyroid controls how quickly the body uses energy; it also makes proteins and controls the body's sensitivity to other hormones. A disruption of the metabolism caused by a disorder of the thyroid after menopause causes problems for the skeletal structure that can bring on osteoporosis. Iodine is required by higher animals for synthesizing thyroid hormones, which contain this element. We should not forget that we are *Homo sapiens* thanks to the two milligrams of iodine provided every day by the thyroid gland. Deficiency of this element affects about two billion people and is the leading preventable cause of intellectual disabilities.

The thyroid controls basic metabolism and cardiac rhythm and governs our ability to adapt. It releases thyroxine and requires the iodine found in food to function. It makes it possible to adapt to changes in the environment such as shifts in temperature, language, and emotional problems. It is a catalyst in the emotional life and in communication. Along with the ovaries and adrenals, it controls energy and its production. Especially in cases of stress syndrome, it meets the body's increased energy requirements and helps it adapt to external changes.

We have four parathyroid glands, usually located on the back of the thyroid gland. They are usually about the size of a grain of rice but may be pea-size. Parathyroid hormone and calcitonin (one of the hormones made by the thyroid gland) have key roles in regulating the amount of calcium in the blood and bones thanks to the secretion of parathyroid hormone (or parathormone, PTH), along with the help of ultraviolet light and vitamin D_3. Calcium is the most important element in our bodies (we use it to control many systems), so calcium is regulated very carefully by the body, and the parathyroid glands control the calcium.

Triiodothyronine (T_3)

When affected by the pituitary hormone TSH, the thyroid gland releases an amino acid–based hormone called thyroxine, or T_4 (because it contains four iodine atoms). T_4 is in turn transformed into triiodothyronine, or T_3 (because it contains three iodine atoms), which on average is five times more active than its precursor. Thyroid hormones increase oxygen consumption and heat production; this is the well-known basal metabolic rate (BMR) that makes it possible to burn calories even when resting. The BMR goes down with age, and close to 75 percent of this decline can be attributed to changes that affect the thyroid hormones and their targets.

The actual level of T_3 suffers a modest decline, in the range of 10 to 20 percent, over the course of an adult's life. On the other hand, as we grow older, the peripheral tissues respond less and less to the solicitations of this hormone. T_3 levels also shrink with

► deficiency or excess of iodine
► low-calorie diets
► high-protein diets
► vegetarian (especially vegan) diets
► overconsumption of green tea
► obesity
► lack of sleep

The Thymus

The thymus is a glandular structure of largely lymphoid tissue that functions in cell-mediated immunity by being the site where T cells develop, T cells being critical to the adaptive immune system. It is composed of two identical lobes and is located anatomically in the anterior superior mediastinum, in front of the heart and behind the sternum. It is part of the lymphatic system and releases thymine. It develops quite rapidly from birth to puberty, the time during which it will produce and store the antibodies necessary for a lifetime. It shrinks in volume in adults but can go back into action if the body requires increased production of antibodies and supervision of the immune system. Because of this, its reflex zone is very important.

The Pancreas

The pancreas is located in the abdominal cavity behind the stomach. It is an endocrine gland producing several important hormones, including insulin and glucagon (hyperglycemic factor), at levels of 80 percent and 20 percent respectively. The role of the digestion hormone insulin is to stimulate the absorption of glucose by the cells. This glucose can either be stored in the form of glycogen or triglycerides, or transformed into energy. If hypoglycemia is an issue, then glucagon steps in. It acts on the absorption of amino acids by the cells and on their transformation into proteins. It is important that the balance of insulin and glucagon remains stable.

The pancreas is also an exocrine gland. Exocrine glands produce and secrete substances onto an epithelial surface by way of a duct (examples of exocrine glands include sweat, salivary, mammary, ceruminous, lacrimal, sebaceous, and mucous glands, as well as the pancreas and liver, which are both endocrine and exocrine glands). In this capacity the pancreas secretes pancreatic juice containing digestive enzymes that assist digestion and absorption of nutrients in the small intestine. These enzymes help to further break down the carbohydrates, proteins, and lipids in the chyme.

The Adrenal Glands

The adrenal glands, found above the kidneys, are made up of two parts that are endocrine in nature: the adrenal cortex and the adrenal medulla. The cortex produces a cholinergic chemical transmitter and numerous hormones such as corticosteroids. This group includes mineral-corticosteroids such as aldosterone, which manages the balance between sodium and potassium salts, retaining sodium and eliminating potassium. The glucocorticoids produced by the adrenals reduce the consumption of glucose in the cells, thereby increasing glycemia. The lower the number of lymphocytes in the blood, the less inflammation there is. The adrenals also play a determinative role in stress situations (hunger, thirst, temperature changes).

Androgens (male hormones) are formed from the synthesis and breakdown of corticoids. A lesser number of female sex hormones are also created. The adrenergic adrenal medulla comes from sympathoblast cells and forms a sympathetic paraganglion. It also produces hormones: noradrenaline and adrenaline, which serve as chemical transmitters for postganglionary sympathetic neurons in the sympathetic nervous system.

DHEA

DHEA (didehydroepiandrosterone) is an important endogenous steroid hormone released by the adrenal glands. It attains high levels around the age of twenty-one, diminishes by 40 percent at the age of forty, and at the age of seventy is little more than a memory. Its beneficial effects are many. They include increased immune-system resistance and protection against viral infections that run the gamut from the common cold to herpes. DHEA also stimulates T cells and reduces the immunosuppression of T cells by hydrocortisone. With its tendency to normalize blood sugar level, DHEA also has an antidiabetic effect. It slows the development of certain forms of cancer (antitumor effect) and works against arteriosclerosis, thus providing protection to the cardiovascular system. DHEA acts through inhibition of the synthesis of fatty acids and cholesterol. It retards aging and slows obesity; it also lowers cholesterol. It can be used (as a supplement) in the treatment of Parkinson's and Alzheimer's. Improved calcium absorption made possible by DHEA makes it possible to reduce bone loss caused by osteoporosis.

To apply the brakes to the loss of DHEA after the age of forty there are a variety of steps that can be taken. In the matter of diet, avoid low-fat foods, sugar, and foods that promote high blood sugar, and eat animal proteins. Contrary to what some health experts have claimed, wild yam has no effect on DHEA. In terms of activity, endurance exercises are helpful, but their results are mediocre after the age of seventy.

Curiously, from a psychological perspective it has been found that controlling, domineering women tend to have higher levels of DHEA.

The pancreas and the adrenal glands are capable of working symbiotically or antagonistically. The adrenaline produced by the adrenal glands and the insulin produced by the pancreas stimulate the release and burning of sugar. Emotional shock, pain, and feelings of fear, anxiety, and stress can throw the adrenal glands off balance, as well as the secretions of the liver, pancreas, thyroid, and so forth, depending on individual heredity. When an injury appears some years later, it can be hard to implement the appropriate treatment. Therefore, knowing the history of the pathological phenomenon is of primary importance.

The Ovaries

Estrogen and progesterone are the two hormones primarily released by the ovaries. Estrogen goes through two principal peaks—just before ovulation, and in the middle of the second phase of the cycle. It maintains and develops female sex organs, promotes tissue growth, and stimulates cellular division, especially in the cells of the mucosal layers of the mouth, nose, skin, uterus, and mammary glands. It encourages bone calcification. Estrogen generates water and salt retention, hence weight increase during peak times. It makes the secretions of the sebaceous glands more fluid and inhibits their secretion during an acne outbreak. It causes lower rates of blood cholesterol and inhibits the formation of arteriosclerosis.

Progesterone is released by the corpus luteum of the ovaries. Its role is to transform the mucous membrane that has been highly developed by estrogen, making it more receptive to possible fertilization and the favorable development of the ovum.

Estrogen and Progesterone

These female hormones are obviously very age-determined. Between the ages of forty-five and fifty-five, and sometimes earlier, the synthesis of estrogen and progesterone by the ovaries dries up. Of course, the ovaries still manufacture a little testosterone, which the body transforms into estradiol, an estrogen, and the adrenal glands produce androstenedione, which is also converted into estradiol, but not enough to make up for the loss of the ovarian synthesis. Besides being age-related, the decline of estrogen is also precipitated by tobacco use and a low-fat diet. As well, the decline of progesterone can be precipitated by a diet that is poor in proteins and calories, by poor cardiovascular health, and by stress.

The Testicles

The testicles produce testosterone as well as minute amounts of female hormones.

Testosterone

The testicles secret the male hormone testosterone from DHEA, which itself is a product of cholesterol. Women synthesize small quantities of testosterone through the peripheral conversion of the androstenedione produced by their ovaries and adrenal glands.

Testosterone is a powerful anabolic substance. It prevents the accumulation of fats, particularly in the region of the abdomen, by inhibiting the activity of the lipoprotein lipase enzyme. Lastly, testosterone mobilizes stored fat by increasing the number of certain adrenergic receptors. The level of testosterone in obese persons exhibiting an excess of abdominal fat is generally low. After reaching its high point in the period between the ages of twenty and thirty, the level of free (available) testosterone in men gradually declines. A man of sixty has two times less testosterone on average than a younger man of twenty-five, and more than 20 percent of the men over sixty have extremely low levels. Even though women have much less testosterone than men, it diminishes the same way in both sexes with age. In addition to its loss being age-related, the level of free testosterone also declines with

▶ low-calorie diets
▶ consumption of soy and its byproducts, legumes, high-fiber foods (whole grains), and flax oil
▶ too much alcohol
▶ exposure to certain pesticides
▶ chronic stress and depression
▶ intense physical effort (as in high-level sports)

To slow down testosterone loss after the age of forty one can take certain steps, beginning with the kind of food eaten. A diet in which 30 percent of the calories ingested are in the form of fat is important, and animal fats should never be entirely removed from the diet. Food supplements can also sometimes help maintain adequate levels of testosterone. Men should take between 5 and 10 milligrams of zinc every day. Physical activities are also helpful, such as those that call for moderate endurance or muscular effort (but their effects can be reduced after age sixty). Sexual activity also stimulates testosterone production. From a psychological standpoint, displaying a somewhat competitive attitude in business and in life can also be helpful.

Related Organs and Systems

In addition to the various specialized endocrine organs, many other organs that are part of other body systems, such as bones, kidneys, liver, and heart, have secondary endocrine functions. For example, the liver secretes insulinlike growth factor (which has insulin effects and regulates growth), angiotensinogen and angiotensin (important in vasoconstriction and the release of aldosterone from adrenal cortex dipsogen), thrombopoietin (which stimulates megakaryocytes to produce platelets), and hepcidin (which inhibits intestinal iron absorption and iron release by macrophages). The heart secretes atrial-natriuretic peptide and brain natriuretic peptide (both important in blood pressure). And the kidneys secrete endocrine hormones such as erythropoietin and renin.

Renin-Angiotensin System (RAS)

The renin-angiotensin system, or RAS, is a hormonal system that regulates blood pressure and fluid balance. When blood pressure goes down, the kidneys release renin, which travels into the bloodstream and triggers the production of angiotensin by the liver. This angiotensin shrinks the diameters of the arteries (vasoconstriction) and thereby raises the blood pressure of the arteries. Angiotensin stimulates the release of aldosterone by the adrenal gland, which increases the amount of salt and water reabsorbed by the kidneys. This process causes elevated blood pressure in the arteries. The control of renin secretion depends on the sodium concentration of the blood, arterial blood pressure, and the action of the sympathetic nervous system.

The Main Organs and Organ Systems

A human organ is a differentiated structure (e.g., a heart or kidney) consisting of cells and tissues that perform some specific function in an organism. When two or more organs work together in the execution of a specific body function they form an organ system (also called a *biological system* or *body system*). The functions of the different organ systems often share significant overlap and are thus studied together, for example, the nervous and endocrine systems (forming the neuroendrocrine system, which we studied in the previous chapter), and the muscular and skeletal systems (forming the musculosketal system), to name just a few.

The Skeletal System

The vitality of a person can be seen in his or her standing posture. The skeleton, that part of the body that supports an organism, goes through profound transformations over the course of a lifetime, particularly at the time of hormonal changes (growing up, puberty, meno-

pause). The bones contains minerals that are, literally, the bricks of the body. The parathyroids, controlled by the liver, set up and adjust the placement of the bones of the skeleton, and the pituitary gland has an effect on bone growth.

Healthy bones require:

► a balanced diet and adequate levels of vitamins C, D, and B
► proper absorption by the intestine
► a well-functioning hormonal system
► regular physical activity, which stimulates the formation of bone cells

A deficient and/or acidic diet (too much sugar, tomatoes, citrus fruits, tea, coffee) is harmful to the bones, as is stress, which blocks the stomach, producing acids that irritate the mucous membrane, making it impermeable to minerals. In the event of a health crisis, meats, fish, and dairy products should be eliminated from the diet.

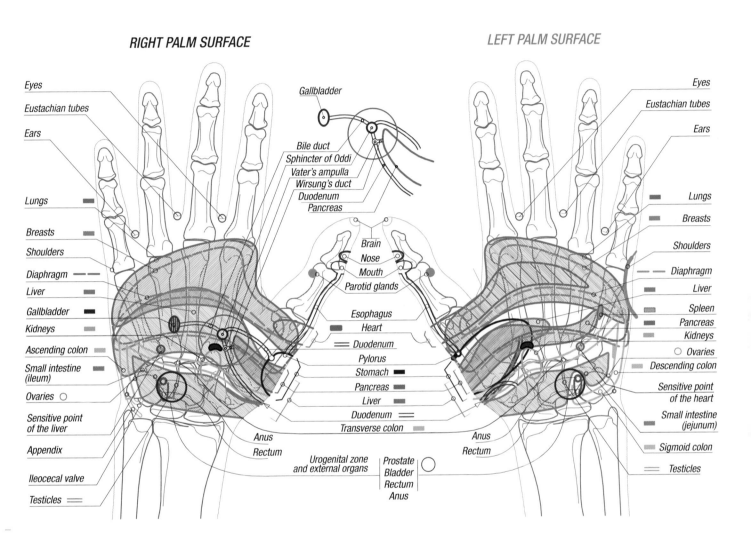

RIGHT PALM SURFACE

LEFT PALM SURFACE

Eyes
Eustachian tubes
Ears

Lungs
Breasts
Shoulders
Diaphragm
Liver
Gallbladder
Kidneys
Ascending colon
Small intestine (ileum)
Ovaries
Sensitive point of the liver
Appendix
Ileocecal valve
Testicles

Gallbladder
Bile duct
Sphincter of Oddi
Vater's ampulla
Wirsung's duct
Duodenum
Pancreas

Brain
Nose
Mouth
Parotid glands
Esophagus
Heart
Duodenum
Pylorus
Stomach
Pancreas
Liver
Duodenum
Transverse colon
Anus
Rectum

Urogenital zone and external organs

Prostate
Bladder
Rectum
Anus

Eyes
Eustachian tubes
Ears
Lungs
Breasts
Shoulders
Diaphragm
Liver
Spleen
Pancreas
Kidneys
Ovaries
Descending colon
Sensitive point of the heart
Small intestine (jejunum)
Sigmoid colon
Testicles

Anus
Rectum

The Digestive System

The digestive system manages food assimilation and eliminates the wastes produced by the digestive process in the stools. It consists of a long tube running through the body from the mouth to the anus. The pelvic parasympathetic system controls the bottom end of the digestive tract (descending colon and rectum). Several kinds of digestive disorders are caused by imbalances in the autonomic nervous system. The pneumogastric nerve innervates all the digestive organs and promotes the digestion and absorption of food.

▶ The mouth and the duodenum transform carbohydrates into glucose.

▶ The stomach transforms proteins into polypeptides; it also reabsorbs iron.

▶ The pancreas digests carbohydrates, lipids, and proteins, and serves a hormonal function.

▶ The duodenum and jejunum break down polypeptides into amino acids. Their digestion of lipids goes through three stages.

▶ The liver digests fats and processes the hormonal steroids, starting with cholesterol. It metabolizes carbohydrates and governs muscle and tendon function.

▶ The bile emulsifies fats.

▶ The pancreas hydrolizes fats.

▶ The mucous membrane of the jejunum then absorbs them.

▶ Lastly, they are transported by the lymph through the thoracic duct to the liver.

▶ The small intestine and colon absorb water and mineral salts.

▶ The jejunum absorbs calcium, and the ileum absorbs vitamins B, C, H, and P.

The Liver

The largest digestive organ in the body and the second biggest organ after the skin, the liver weighs more than three pounds. Oval-shaped, it is located beneath the diaphragm on the right side of the abdominal cavity, strategically placed within the circulatory system. It is irrigated by the portal vein from the entire intestinal tract, which is rich in nutrients, and the inferior vena cava, from the heart, which is rich in oxygen. A vascular reddish brown in color, it filters 1.5 liters of blood each minute, which amounts to 90 liters an hour, or 2,160 liters a day. Made up of specialized epithelial cells that form lobes called *hepatocytes,* the liver controls the various forms of metabolism in the body. For this reason the liver works with other organs and anatomical systems: the brain, kidneys, heart, bones, endocrine system, immune system, and so forth.

The liver is a veritable factory of biochemical transformations, an excretory system that performs both exocrine and endocrine functions. Its major role is to metabolize, detoxify, and deactivate endogenous and exogenous compounds that have no nutritional value. It performs more than five hundred integrated vital functions. It is extremely sensitive and reacts to emotions that affect a person's integrity and sense of oneness (the deep self).

Vascular function: filtering of the blood

Metabolic functions: metabolism of carbohydrates (storage of glycogens, maintenance of stable blood sugar levels); conversion of galactose and fructose into glucose; glycogenolysis (in cases of acute stress, as in the fight-or-flight response); neoglucogenesis (in cases of chronic stress)

Metabolizing of fats: oxidation of fatty acids (production of energy in the form of ATP); formation of lipoproteins (transport of cholesterol and steroidal hormones); production of cholesterol, triglycerides, and phospholipids (cellular membrane, adipocytes, and biliary salts); conversion of carbohydrates and proteins into fats, storage of energy reserves

Metabolism of proteins: production of ATP, a coenzyme used as an energy carrier (or conversion of arachidonic acid, AA, or ARA into carbohydrates or lipids); plasma production (alpha and beta globulins, prothrombin, fibrinogens, and albumin); conversion of ammonia (NH_3) into urea, excreted in urine; storage of vitamins A, B, D, E, K, and B_{12}); storage of the minerals iron and copper

Secreting and excreting functions: formation, storage in gallbladder, and excretion of bile at a rate of 800 to 1000 ml daily; production of the active form of vitamin D

The Liver's Detoxifying Functions

Clearly, one of the main functions of the liver is detoxification. The transformation and elimination of toxic substances from the body, as found in phase 1 and phase 2 detoxification, is critical for understanding the profound implications of inflammation and chronic diseases. Other specific detoxification functions of the liver include:

▶ the catabolism of steroid and thyroid hormones
▶ the phagocytosis (destruction) of worn-out red and white blood corpuscles and disease-causing bacteria (neutrophil-Kupffer cells help eliminate bacteria in the liver)
▶ the production of bile for the elimination of metabolic wastes like bilirubin and cholesterol, and for the promotion of digestion and the absorption of lipids

The liver also converts important vitamins and hormones into more active forms, as in the hydroxylation of vitamin D and its deiodination (removal of iodine) into T_4 and T_3.

Hepatotoxicity

Hepatocytes make up 70 to 85 percent of the liver's mass. These cells are involved in protein synthesis and storage; transformation of carbohydrates; synthesis of cholesterol, bile salts, and phospholipids; detoxification, modification, and excretion of exogenous and endogenous substances; and initiation of formation and secretion of bile. Hepatocytes are the preferred target of the toxins present in the chemical poisoning of the environment. This chemical-driven toxicity causes liver damage.

Every substance that is foreign to the organism's physiology is called *xenobiotic.* There are two classes of xenobiotics: exogenous (including various chemical products and some plants, mushrooms, and antifoods like ethanol) and endogenous (the natural wastes created by cellular metabolism or by the bacteria of the intestinal flora). Xenobiotic substances are able to gain entry into the body by ways of the digestive system, the pulmonary system, and the skin. The largest pathway for hepatic toxicity, which alters the function and structure of hepatocytes and their organelles, is most likely the gastrointestinal tract. Oral exogenous xenobiotic substances travel directly into the liver through the portal system in the company of the nutrients that have been absorbed. As they are not cellular nutrients, xenobiotic substances are discharged into the duodenum by means of bile movement, which itself is produced by the canicular membranes of the hepatocytes, hence the enterohepatic circulation.

The structure of xenobiotic substances makes them hydrophobic, which entails their biochemical transformation through metabolic oxidation into hydrophilic substances for the purpose of expelling them from the body by way of the renal or intestinal systems.

The Respiratory System

The respiratory system consists of the lungs and the bronchial tubes. The lungs are wrapped in the pleura and are entirely protected within the thoracic cavity. These are the organs of breath, as in "the breath of life." During intrauterine life and at the moment of birth, a baby's lungs are full of water. It is only after the umbilical cord has been cut that they fill with air. This causes the baby to howl. A newborn human being thus begins life with the beginning of the inhalation/exhalation cycle that will last for the duration of that being's lifetime.

A few other facts about the respiratory system:

▶ Respiratory rhythm consists of an average of fourteen inhalations and exhalations per minute.
▶ Along with diet, the lungs are the source of vital energy for the body.
▶ Along with the nose and trachea, the lungs and bronchial tubes are the first ramparts against airborne assaults from the environment (pollution).

The Pleurae

The walls of the pleurae, the delicate serous membranes that line each half of the thorax and are folded back over the surface of the lungs, must be perfectly smooth both inside and out. Between the two layers of pleura the pressure is negative in order to keep the lungs dilated and to help the heart suck up the blood of the veins. To ensure that the pleurae continue to function optimally they must be protected from smoke, dust, and other particulate matter, as well as from physical trauma to the spinal column and ribs.

Every day we breathe in and out around 2,100 times, while some 2,300 gallons (9,000 liters) of air enter and leave our lungs daily, more than the capacity of the average tanker truck! It is the cerebral bulb located just above the spinal cord that governs the respiratory cycle by activating the diaphragm.

Many people think that when they breathe they are inhaling only oxygen. In fact, we are breathing in 79 percent nitrogen and 21 percent oxygen along with water vapor and some rare gases like helium. Obviously, only the oxygen is essential, and the 21 percent that is absorbed is entirely needed. Respiration is affected by the amount of carbon dioxide in the blood. An abnormal increase of carbon dioxide in the bloodstream can lead to asphyxiation.

The Bronchial Tubes, an Exchange Network

The multiple branches that extend from the bronchioles (the minute, thin-walled branch of the bronchae) to the aleveoli (the terminal ends of the respiratory tree, which outcrop from either alveolar sacs or alveolar ducts, which are both sites of gas exchange with the blood, and of which we have close to 300 million) make the circulation of air possible in the lungs. They produce a liter of secretions a day intended to keep the lungs moist and to evacuate impurities. These secretions are discharged directly into the digestive tract.

When the respiratory system is not functioning very well, the first consequence is difficulty in breathing normally. Inhalation and exhalation can be loud. Fatigue, lack of vigor, and back pain in the region of the shoulder blades accompany respiratory inadequacy. Outbursts of bad temper can be explained by an excess of carbon dioxide in the bloodstream. The person may easily become out of breath when making any sort of effort. The heart beats faster and the pulse is rapid. A stitch in the side is a common occurrence, and there can be excessive perspiration.

The Circulatory System

The circulatory system is the network of blood, blood vessels, lymphatics, and the heart concerned with the circulation of the blood and lymph. The heart propels blood from its left region into the major circulatory arterial vessels and from there to the peripheral capillaries. The blood returns to the right side of the heart through the vein network, where it is then propelled from the right ventricle to the lungs, from where it returns to the left side. This is known as pulmonary, or minor, circulation.

The heart is the first organ of the human body to function. It begins beating during the third week of the embryo's life; it is the last organ to stop at death.

▶ Cardiac output is 1.3 gallons (5 liters) a minute, and the heart beats seventy times during that period of time.

▶ Every day the heart expels 1,900 gallons (7,200 liters) of blood (the body holds between 1.3 and 1.8 gallons, or 5 to 7 liters).

▶ Only the brain requires more oxygen than the heart. The heart gets the oxygen it needs to function properly from the coronary arteries that surround the heart.

▶ The coronary arteries transmit around 95 gallons (360 liters) of blood to the heart daily when resting. When the diameter of these major arteries is reduced by stenosis or cholesterol build-up, this deprives the heart of oxygen, which poses a major risk of heart attack.

Cardiac rhythm is directly influenced by worry and stress, which means that the emotions target us directly in the heart. The "lump in one's throat" is literally the heart's response to great emotions or to deep disappointment. Thus a "broken heart" is not merely a metaphor. To listen to a client or a patient with your heart—that is, with compassion and empathy in order to find just the right words—is the panacea of any therapy, providing relief and relaxation of tension.

High Blood Pressure

Blood pressure is the pressure exerted by the blood on the walls of the blood vessels and especially the arteries. It is expressed as a fraction having as a numerator the maximum pressure that follows the cardiac systole (the contraction of the heart by which the blood is forced onward and the circulation kept up) of the left ventricle of the heart, and as a denominator the minimum pressure that accompanies cardiac diastole (the passive rhythmical expansion or dilation of the cavities of the heart during which they fill with blood). According to the American Heart Association, normal blood pressure in an adult is 120/80. Blood pressure is considered high when it goes above 140/90; this indicates sympatheticotonia, a stimulated condition of the sympathetic nervous system marked by vascular spasm, heightened blood pressure, and the dominance of other functions of the sympathetic nervous system.

Certain factors (stress, tobacco use, overeating, pharmaceutical use, birth control pills) make the bed of arteriosclerosis, the thickening, hardening, and loss of elasticity of the walls of arteries, which is a significant health risk. High blood pressure can also have hereditary, family, hormonal, and renal causes.

The Circulatory System
Veins and Arteries

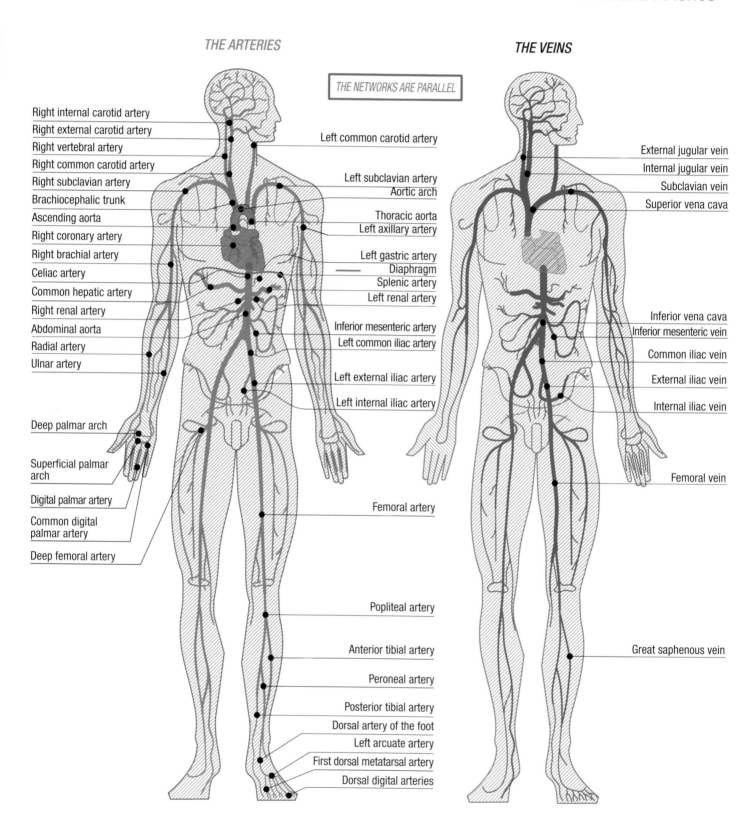

THE ARTERIES

THE VEINS

THE NETWORKS ARE PARALLEL

Right internal carotid artery
Right external carotid artery
Right vertebral artery
Right common carotid artery
Right subclavian artery
Brachiocephalic trunk
Ascending aorta
Right coronary artery
Right brachial artery
Celiac artery
Common hepatic artery
Right renal artery
Abdominal aorta
Radial artery
Ulnar artery

Deep palmar arch

Superficial palmar arch

Digital palmar artery

Common digital palmar artery

Deep femoral artery

Left common carotid artery

Left subclavian artery
Aortic arch

Thoracic aorta
Left axillary artery

Left gastric artery
Diaphragm
Splenic artery
Left renal artery

Inferior mesenteric artery
Left common iliac artery

Left external iliac artery

Left internal iliac artery

Femoral artery

Popliteal artery

Anterior tibial artery

Peroneal artery

Posterior tibial artery
Dorsal artery of the foot
Left arcuate artery
First dorsal metatarsal artery
Dorsal digital arteries

External jugular vein
Internal jugular vein
Subclavian vein
Superior vena cava

Inferior vena cava
Inferior mesenteric vein

Common iliac vein

External iliac vein

Internal iliac vein

Femoral vein

Great saphenous vein

The Circulatory System
Reflex Points

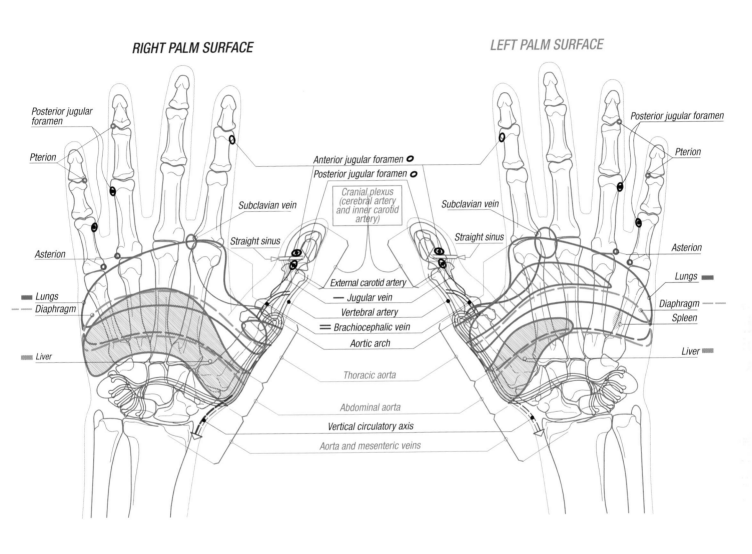

RIGHT PALM SURFACE

LEFT PALM SURFACE

Posterior jugular foramen

Pterion

Subclavian vein

Straight sinus

Asterion

Lungs
Diaphragm

Liver

Anterior jugular foramen
Posterior jugular foramen

Cranial plexus
(cerebral artery
and inner carotid
artery)

External carotid artery
Jugular vein
Vertebral artery
Brachiocephalic vein
Aortic arch

Thoracic aorta

Abdominal aorta

Vertical circulatory axis

Aorta and mesenteric veins

Posterior jugular foramen

Pterion

Subclavian vein

Straight sinus

Asterion

Lungs

Diaphragm
Spleen

Liver

Synthesis of the Digestive and Circulatory Systems

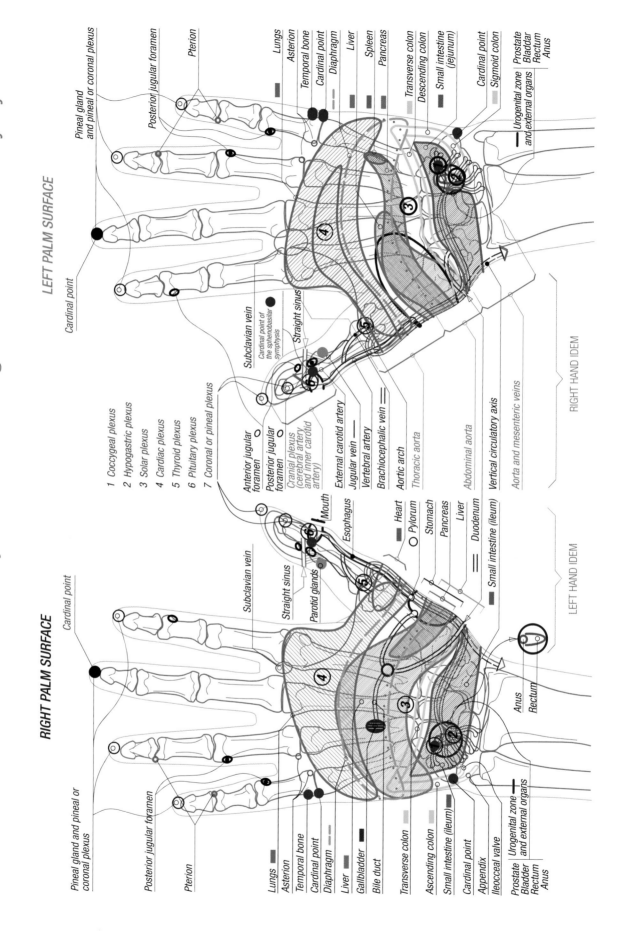

LEFT PALM SURFACE

Cardinal point

Pineal gland and pineal or coronal plexus

Posterior jugular foramen

Pterion

Lungs
Asterion
Temporal bone
Cardinal point
Diaphragm
Liver
Spleen
Pancreas

Transverse colon
Descending colon

Small intestine (jejunum)

Cardinal point
Sigmoid colon

Urogenital zone and external organs

Prostate
Bladdar
Rectum
Anus

Subclavian vein
Cardinal point of the sphenobasilar symphysis
Straight sinus

Anterior jugular foramen
Posterior jugular foramen
Cranial plexus (cerebral artery and inner carotid artery)

External carotid artery
Jugular vein
Vertebral artery
Brachiocephalic vein
Aortic arch
Thoracic aorta

Abdominal aorta

Vertical circulatory axis

Aorta and mesenteric veins

RIGHT HAND IDEM

1 Coccygeal plexus
2 Hypogastric plexus
3 Solar plexus
4 Cardiac plexus
5 Thyroid plexus
6 Pituitary plexus
7 Coronal or pineal plexus

RIGHT PALM SURFACE

Cardinal point

Subclavian vein
Straight sinus
Parotid glands

Mouth
Esophagus

Heart
Pylorum
Stomach
Pancreas
Liver
Duodenum

Small intestine (ileum)

LEFT HAND IDEM

Anus
Rectum

Pineal gland and pineal or coronal plexus

Posterior jugular foramen

Pterion

Lungs
Asterion
Temporal bone
Cardinal point
Diaphragm
Liver
Gallbladder
Bile duct

Transverse colon
Ascending colon
Small intestine (ileum)
Cardinal point
Appendix
Ileocceal valve

Urogenital zone and external organs

Prostate
Bladder
Rectum
Anus

82 ◆ Hand Reflexology and the Systems and Energy Centers of the Body

Synthesis of the Points of the Cardiorespiratory and Circulatory Systems

LEFT PALM SURFACE

RIGHT PALM SURFACE

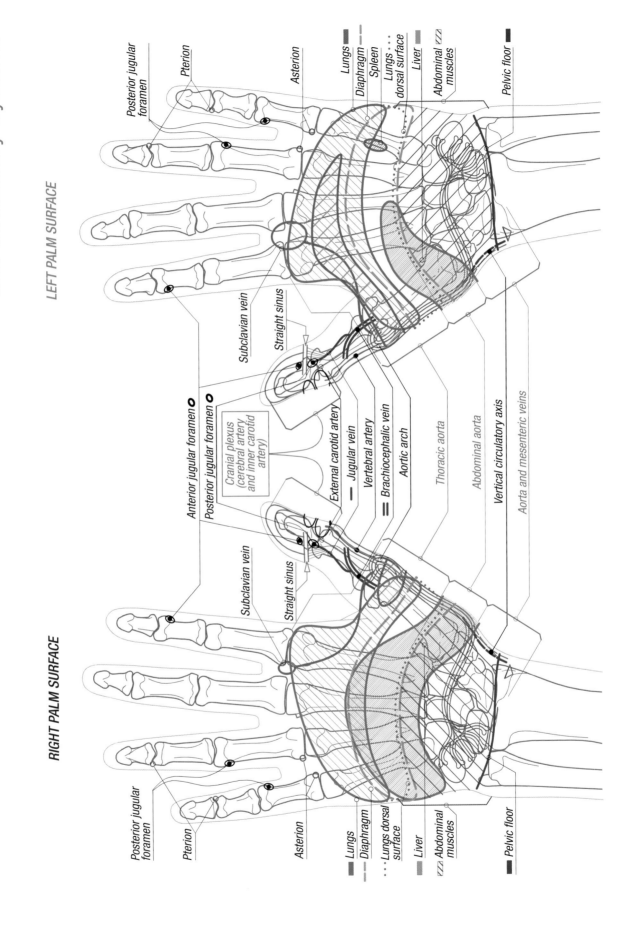

Posterior jugular foramen

Pterion

Asterion

Lungs
Diaphragm
Spleen
Lungs · · · dorsal surface
Liver
Abdominal muscles
Pelvic floor

Subclavian vein

Straight sinus

Anterior jugular foramen
Posterior jugular foramen

Cranial plexus (cerebral artery and inner carotid artery)

External carotid artery
Jugular vein
Vertebral artery
Brachiocephalic vein
Aortic arch

Thoracic aorta

Abdominal aorta

Vertical circulatory axis

Aorta and mesenteric veins

Subclavian vein

Straight sinus

Posterior jugular foramen

Pterion

Asterion

Lungs
Diaphragm
Lungs dorsal surface
Liver
Abdominal muscles
Pelvic floor

The Immune System

Unlike other bodily systems, the immune system is not made up of specific groups of physical structures. Rather, it consists of the complex interactions between different organs and substances of the different organs, and the multiple functions they perform. The immune system protects the body from foreign substances, cells, and tissues by producing an immune response that includes the thymus, spleen, lymph nodes, special deposits of lymphoid tissue (as in the gastrointestinal tract and bone marrow), lymphocytes (including B cells and T cells), and antibodies, which serve to destroy or neutralize foreign substances or infectious disease organisms.

The immune system relies on the balanced function of the liver, spleen, intestines, and autonomic nervous system. When a profound stress has not been fully integrated, the body falls into a sympathicotonic state that causes a continuous release of adrenaline, which then produces sleep disorders, fatigue, weight loss, and poor digestion. This has an echo effect on the body's entire glandular system, with the immune system particularly affected. The irritable or depressed mood that stress causes leads to one of two responses: the person will either recognize what is happening and allow his or her body to enter a parasympathicotonic state; or he or she will not see the warning signal for what it is and continue to force the body to keep going, like whipping a recalcitrant horse, with an increasing reliance on stimulants like coffee, tobacco, alcohol, and psychotropic drugs. And so whereas becoming conscious of a stress creates a positive response and consequently a physical reaction that promotes good immune function, ignoring stress causes a negative response that in turn makes the body more vulnerable. When the immune system is weakened, even minor viruses or bacteria, innocuous under ordinary circumstances, can wreak havoc. Weakening of the immune system increases the vulnerability of the nervous system and the hormonal system and makes it possible for many different diseases to get a foothold in the body.

The principal signs of poor immune system function or a compromised immune system include:

- ▶ excessive, persistent fatigue
- ▶ hyperactivity, agitation
- ▶ repeated infections
- ▶ multiple cases of inflammation
- ▶ allergies
- ▶ wounds, injuries, or infections that are slow to heal
- ▶ chronic diarrhea
- ▶ oral or genital herpes
- ▶ chronic infection of the mucous membranes
- ▶ colds, persistent coughs
- ▶ frequent vaginal and various kinds of fungal infections

When the body is in poor health, conventional medicine goes to war against disease using pharmaceutical medications, radiation, and invasive surgery in an attempt to restore the balance that is the indispensable property of true health. This balance can never be truly restored unless the immune system has been revitalized, allowing the body to come to a natural state of homeostasis.

Understanding what a well-functioning immune system consists of is essential for taking care of oneself as well as one's clients and patients. A reflexology treatment should integrate the various immune system components that are liable to come into play in order to help the body promote a better immune response.

The strength of the immune system varies according to age, sex, genetic factors, and nutrition. Babies possess a natural immune system but their acquired immunity to specific diseases comes from the antibodies provided by the mother during the first six months of nursing. Before menopause, women have much more effective immune systems than men because of their extremely active hormonal cycles. The immune defenses of the elderly are weaker than those of younger people because lymphocytes take longer to mature the older we become.

Fever and inflammation actually have a beneficial effect on the natural immune system because they increase the migration of microphages, stimulating the antiviral activities of interferons. Natural therapies like homeopathy respect the vital evolution of these symptoms, and instead of bringing them to an abrupt halt they guide their effects for the benefit of the person.

A deficient genetic makeup or poor diet weakens the body's natural immune system. Other threats are posed by stress and emotional trauma, which stimulates the adrenal-hypthalamopituitary axis. This results in an excessive production of adrenaline, glucagons, and cortisol, which elevate blood sugar and are anti-inflammatory. They also raise blood pressure. It is important to keep this process in mind when treating chronic diseases or working with people who have been subjected to longstanding, recurring stressors.

The skin, which forms a barrier, and sweat, whose moderate acidity protects the digestive, nasopharyngeal, and urogenital membranes, make up the immune system's first line of defense. Supporting roles are played by phagocytes, which eat harmful foreign particles, bacteria, and dead or dying cells and which are natural antibiotics; and interferons, which are proteins made and released by host cells in response to the presence of pathogens such as viruses, bacteria, parasites, and tumor cells.

Deficiencies in zinc and vitamins C and B, as well as excessive consumption of animal proteins, can weaken the natural immune system.

The Two Branches of the Immune System

The immune system is in place from the moment of birth. It only functions partially at this time because it is still immature and must learn to defend itself against outside invaders called *antigens*. It first has to learn to identify then to remember certain specific antigens that it encountered earlier. This aptitude is the work of both branches of the immune system: cell-mediated immunity and humoral immunity.

In humoral immunity, the protective function of immunization is mediated by macromolecules found in bodily fluids such as secreted antibodies, complement proteins, and certain antimicrobial peptides. These are not cells, but rather special proteins whose chemical structure is designed to allow them to be applied to the surface of certain specific antigens in a way that is similar to their structure. When these proteins encounter their specific antigen targets, the antibodies destroy the enemy cells or alert the white cells, which in turn attack the intruder antigens.

Antibodies are produced by another group of white cells, B lymphocytes, which are produced by the bone marrow. When B lymphocytes are introduced to a particular antigen, they program an antibody that adjusts itself to glue over the intruder antigen perfectly. It also records the identity of the invader in order to prompt the manufacture of similar antibodies in case this same antigen makes an appearance in the future. For this system to work, each new cell is programmed so it can produce an infinite variety of antibodies intended to recognize, then copy and adhere to, any kind of antigen it encounters. This mechanism is known as *jumping genes*. Inside B cells, the gene responsible for the chemical structure of the protein it will produce can be freely altered and bonded in accordance with numerous combinations. Every cell is thereby capable of producing an antibody molecule that has the ability to recognize and "copy" any invader. It is humoral immunity that makes vaccination possible.

In cell-mediated, or cellular immunity, the protective function of immunization is associated with cells. The white cells known as T cells are the ones that identify or destroy cancer cells, viruses, bacteria, and fungi. T cells mature in the thymus. These T cells (or T lymphocytes) learn how to recognize the "self" that must be tolerated and the "nonself" that must be destroyed. The thymus is located behind the sternum and is the major gland of the immune system. T cells are programmed in the thymus to recognize and identify a special form of enemy invader. Not all T cells survive the trial period in the thymus. Those that are not programmed perfectly are rejected, for example, if they are unable to make the distinction between what is the self and what is the nonself. The cells that pass this text successfully are discharged into the bloodstream to recognize and destroy the antigens corresponding to their initial programming. They attack these antigens by secreting proteins called *cytokines,* the best known of which is interferon.

White Blood Cells

White blood cells (WBCs) are the principal operating cells of the immune system, so named because of the physical appearance of a blood sample after centrifugation. WBCs are involved in protecting the body against both infectious disease and foreign invaders. All leukocytes are produced and derived from a multipotent cell in the bone marrow known as a *hematopoietic stem cell.* Leukocytes are found throughout the body, including the blood and lymphatic system. White blood cells are larger than red ones; they can move independently in the bloodstream and can cross through the cellular membrane no matter what their size. They are therefore able to travel more quickly to an infected site. There are several categories of WBCs, each of which has its own specific function.

Granulocytes

Granulocytes are a category of white blood cells characterized by the presence of granules in their cytoplasm. There are three kinds of granulocytes:

Neutrophils: These are by far the most abundant. Their purpose is to ingest and destroy microorganisms and bacteria.

Eosinophils: These ingest and destroy the antibody/antigen combinations and modify allergic and hypersensitive reactions by releasing an enzyme that shrinks the histamine molecule so that it can be absorbed. People with allergies have a large quantity of eosinophils in their bloodstreams.

Basophils: These granulocyte cells release heparin or histamine in response to contact with an antigen.

Lymphocytes

There are three kinds of this subtype of white blood cell:

T cells: These cells originate in the bone marrow, mature in the thymus, and play a major role in cell-mediated immunity.

B cells: These cells originate in the bone marrow and are responsible for the production of antibodies.

Natural killer cells (NK cells): Their mission is to destroy infected cells or those that have become cancerous.

Monocytes

This subtype of WBC is the largest in the body. The job of monocytes is to gather together the wastes produced by the body. They store and digest the particles that must be destroyed, such as aging cells, tumor cells, and so forth. In this capacity they are known as *macrophages* when they are in the tissues, where they perform the same functions as when they are in the bloodstream.

The Lymphatic System

There is another important player in the immune system: the lymphatic system. This consists of various organs: the spleen, thymus, tonsils, and lymph nodes. Lymph, a clear fluid (from Latin *lympha,* "water"), circulates through the the lymphatic vessels that are part of the circulatory system and bathes every cell of the body. It should be noted that *the cell breathes in the lymph and the lymph breathes in the blood.* Lymph is produced by the interstitial milieu in which all exchanges ensuring the life of the cells occur. Cells draw from lymph the elements they need to survive and expel into it combustion residues. The lymphatic capillaries originate in the interstitial space. With a cellular structure that is looser than that of the venules (any of the minute veins connecting the capillaries with the larger systemic veins), they are able to reabsorb the proteins and lipids whose molecular weight is too high to permit them back into the venules.

The lymphatic system operates as the principal cleanser of the cells. Extracellular fluid is transported through the lymphatic system, carrying with it all the toxins produced by the metabolism. Lymph travels through the lymph nodes in which live the macrophages that filter out all undesirable substances. Once the lymph has been cleansed, it goes back into the bloodstream.

During an infection, lymphocytes multiply in the lymphoid follicles to neutralize the invading antigens. The thymus, which is located in the mediastinum and has a tendency to atrophy in adults, manufactures these lymphocytes. It plays a major role in the body's fight against cancer. The spleen is also a lymphoid organ. It filters the blood, recovers iron from red blood cells that have become too old, stores lymphocytes, and in certain metabolic disorders stores large quantities of fat. The tonsils, adenoids, the ileocecal valve (the connection between the small and large intestines), and the appendix all have lymphoid tissue. Lymphoid follicles can also be found in the liver and the mucous membrane of the intestines. This latter is known as GALT, "gut-associated lymphatic tissue."

The lymphatic system, marvelous as it is, cannot work properly if it is not well-maintained with a supply of good nutrients. A number of dietary substances support lymph node function and prevent disease. Polyunsaturated fatty acids as found in nuts, seeds, fish, and whole grains, as well as dairy products, tofu, and leafy greens, which are natural sources of vitamin D, can potentially help preserve healthy lymph nodes.

On the other hand, numerous environmental factors affect the lymphatic system and compromise the balance of the immune system. It is therefore important to take all the necessary steps to avoid situations that pose a danger of weakening it. This includes exposure to chemical household products, pesticides, pollutants, food additives, antibiotics, pharmaceutical drugs, and so forth.

Connective Tissue

Connective tissue (also known as *conjunctive tissue*) is of primary importance not only in lymphatic exchanges but also in nerve exchanges circulatory exchanges, and in the apportionment of cerebrospinal fluid. The balance of the overall circulation is maintained by the blood circulation by means of arterioles (any of the small terminal twigs of an artery that ends in capillaries) and venoles. These smaller vessels are therefore of greater importance than the larger vessels, as they guarantee the balance of the entire circulatory system.

Cells of the immune system such as macrophages, mast cells, plasma cells, and eosinophils are found scattered in loose connective tissue, providing the ground for starting inflammatory and immune responses upon the detection of antigens.

Cerebrospinal Fluid (CSF)

Cerebrospinal fluid, a clear, colorless body fluid found in the brain and spine, plays an essential role in the immune system because of the antibodies it transports. It acts as a cushion or buffer for the brain's cortex, providing basic mechanical and immunological protection to the brain inside the skull. The CSF also serves a vital function in cerebral autoregulation of cerebral blood flow. A blockage caused by physical, emotional, or spiritual whiplash slows the circulation of the cerebrospinal fluid, thereby weakening the body's immune system and therefore the body's resistance to disease.

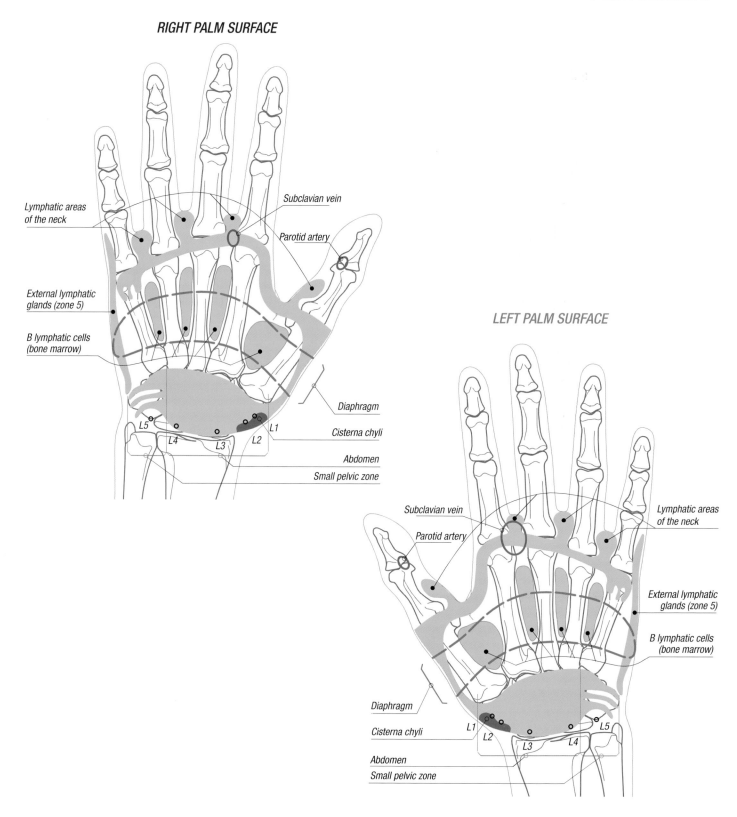

RIGHT PALM SURFACE

Lymphatic areas
of the neck

Subclavian vein

Parotid artery

External lymphatic
glands (zone 5)

B lymphatic cells
(bone marrow)

Diaphragm

Cisterna chyli

Abdomen

Small pelvic zone

L5 L4 L3 L2 L1

LEFT PALM SURFACE

Subclavian vein

Parotid artery

Lymphatic areas
of the neck

External lymphatic
glands (zone 5)

B lymphatic cells
(bone marrow)

Diaphragm

Cisterna chyli

Abdomen

Small pelvic zone

L1 L2 L3 L4 L5

RIGHT DORSAL SURFACE

LEFT DORSAL SURFACE

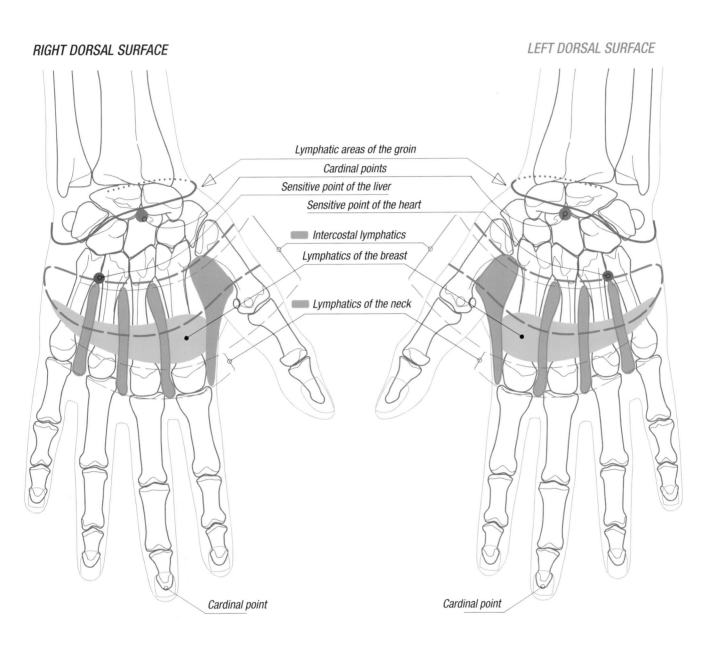

Lymphatic areas of the groin

Cardinal points

Sensitive point of the liver

Sensitive point of the heart

Intercostal lymphatics

Lymphatics of the breast

Lymphatics of the neck

Cardinal point

Cardinal point

INNER LATERAL

*Circular reflex treatment
(three times around)*

Treatment path on the inner surface · · · · · · · ·
Treatment path on the outer surface ————

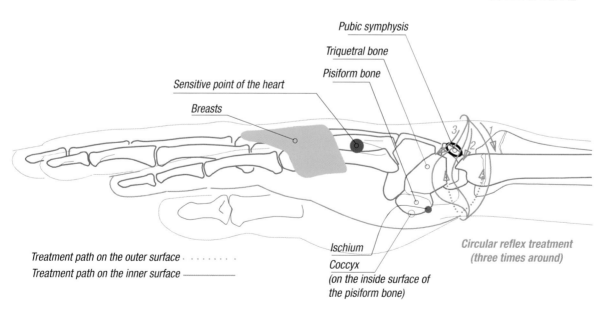

Pecquet's cistern

Thymus

Thyroid

Tonsils

Submandibular glands

OUTER LATERAL

Pubic symphysis

Triquetral bone

Pisiform bone

Sensitive point of the heart

Breasts

Ischium

Coccyx
(on the inside surface of
the pisiform bone)

Treatment path on the outer surface · · · · · · · ·
Treatment path on the inner surface ————

*Circular reflex treatment
(three times around)*

Circulation of the Cerebrospinal Fluid

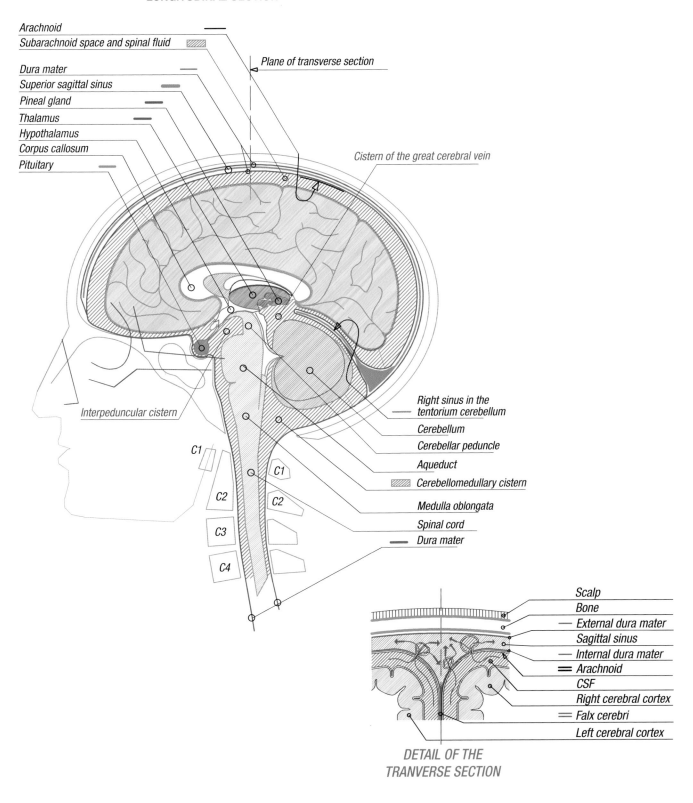

LONGITUDINAL SECTION

Arachnoid
Subarachnoid space and spinal fluid

Dura mater
Superior sagittal sinus
Pineal gland
Thalamus
Hypothalamus
Corpus callosum
Pituitary

Plane of transverse section

Cistern of the great cerebral vein

Interpeduncular cistern

C1

C1

C2

C2

C3

C4

Right sinus in the tentorium cerebellum
Cerebellum
Cerebellar peduncle
Aqueduct
Cerebellomedullary cistern
Medulla oblongata
Spinal cord
Dura mater

Scalp
Bone
External dura mater
Sagittal sinus
Internal dura mater
Arachnoid
CSF
Right cerebral cortex
Falx cerebri
Left cerebral cortex

*DETAIL OF THE
TRANVERSE SECTION*

The Urinary System

The urinary system is quite an impressive machine. The kidneys, which are essential to the urinary system, filter approximately 48 gallons (180 liters) of blood a day. They produce around 1.5 quarts (1.5 liters) of urine during this same twenty-four-hour period, and the majority of the fluids crossing through their 1,200,000 nephrons, the urine-producing functional structures of the kidney, is reabsorbed by the extracellular terrain.

The Kidneys

The kidneys manage the water of our bodies as well as control blood volume and blood pressure. They ensure that there are proper amounts of sodium, potassium, calcium, phosphate, and bicarbonate in our bodies. They eliminate our wastes. When kidney function is poor, there is a risk of edema. The kidneys also eliminate the wastes and toxins produced by our cells. It could be said that the kidneys, along with the liver, are the great purifiers of our body. They transform proteins (the bulk of which come from meat and cheese) into urea and uric acid. They excrete certain soluble wastes like nitrogen wastes, hormones, and medications. They manufacture some hormones like renin, which has an effect on blood pressure. They also play a role in the synthesis of prostaglandin, which has an effect on the uterus, the digestive system, the bronchia, and pain. Other kidney functions include the stimulation of red blood cell and vitamin D formation, and they make the preservation of glucose possible.

The left kidney and genital system share a large portion of their venous and lymphatic circulation. They are so intimately connected that if one wishes to affect one, the other system must also be involved. This explains why the left kidney is connected to sexuality. Because the venous system of the genital organs is closely related to the left kidney, any genital infection will also have repercussions on the left kidney.

The right kidney is more a dependent of the digestive system. Located beneath the liver, it often combines forces with it and also serves the liver as an overflow reservoir. When both the right kidney and liver are functioning poorly at the same time the body is no longer be able to compensate for this excess. At such times the person will feel extremely tired and quite irritable.

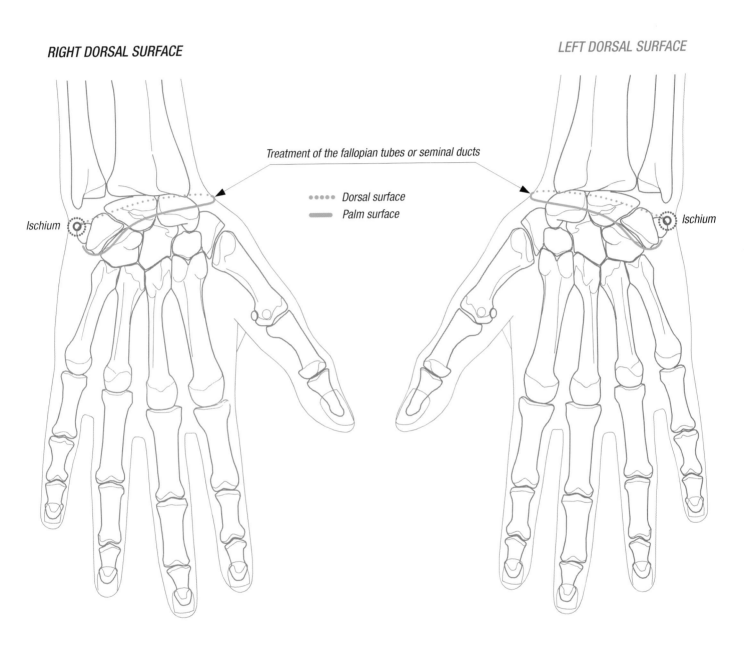

RIGHT DORSAL SURFACE

LEFT DORSAL SURFACE

Treatment of the fallopian tubes or seminal ducts

••••• Dorsal surface
⸻ Palm surface

Ischium

Ischium

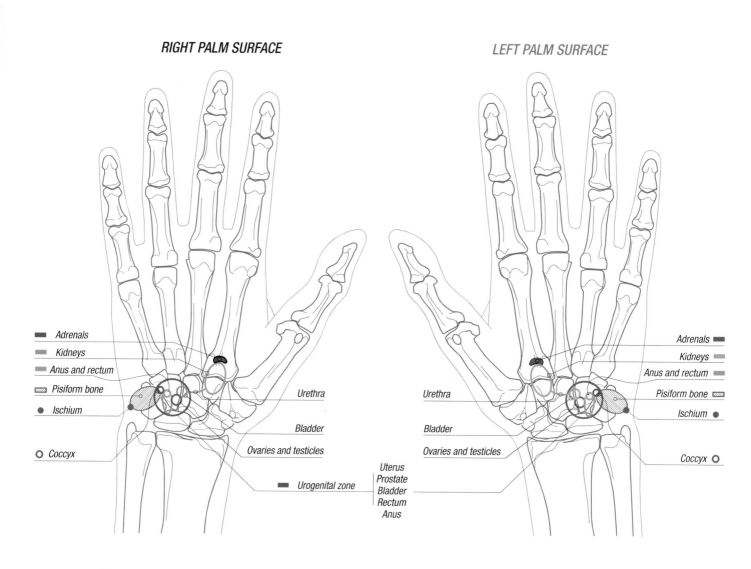

RIGHT PALM SURFACE

LEFT PALM SURFACE

Adrenals

Kidneys

Anus and rectum

Pisiform bone

Ischium

Coccyx

Urethra

Bladder

Ovaries and testicles

Urogenital zone

Uterus
Prostate
Bladder
Rectum
Anus

Urethra

Bladder

Ovaries and testicles

Adrenals

Kidneys

Anus and rectum

Pisiform bone

Ischium

Coccyx

The Plexuses

A *plexus* is a network of interconnecting or interlacing blood vessels or nerves. The plexuses establish contact between the three levels of a person—mental, emotional, and physical—through the brain, endocrine glands, and the cells. The endocrine glands assimilate hormonal signals (the holistic mechanism of integration) and release hormones that are transported by the bloodstream into the cells. Each endocrine center thereby plays a role in the body's physiology and that of each plexus.

The plexuses, of which there are seven, form a kind of crossroads where there is an anastomosis—a union of parts or branches—of the nerves.

▶ On the physical level we have (1) the coccygeal plexus, and (2) the hypogastric plexus.

▶ On the emotional level we have (3) the solar (or digestive) plexus, (4) the cardiac plexus, and (5) the thyroid plexus.

▶ On the mental level there is (6) the pituitary (or hypophyseal) plexus and (7) the pineal (or coronal) plexus.

The Coccygeal Plexus: Procreation, Growth, and Sexuality

This plexus, located near the pubis, can be found on the hand on the lower inside portion of the pisiform bone, a small knobby, pea-shaped bone that is found in the wrist, which forms the ulnar border of the carpal tunnel. It is the seat of procreation, growth, and sexuality.

The testicles release endogens like testosterone, while the ovaries release estrogen and progesterone, which prepares the uterus for implantation. Progesterone also plays an important role in brain function as a neurosteroid. These substances are responsible for secondary sexual characteristics and are involved in the function of the central nervous system and the libido.

The reflexology treatment of this plexus helps regulate growth, sexuality (especially in cases of sterility or loss of libido), and disrupted menstrual cycles.

The Hypogastric Plexus: Elimination and Excretion

This plexus is located two fingers' width beneath the navel, and its reflex point can be found on the hand—palm side up—on the inner edge of the triquetral bone, which is located in the wrist on the medial side of the proximal row of the carpus between the lunate and pisiform bones. It is on the ulnar side of the hand, but it does not articulate with the ulna. It connects with the pisiform, hamate, and lunate bones. This is the seat of elimination and excretion. Bones, nails, and hair draw their energy from this plexus. It is also the seat of creative inspiration. Its corresponding glands are the adrenals.

Reflexology treatment of this point is effective in relieving pain and for dealing with elimination problems and inflammation.

The Plexuses

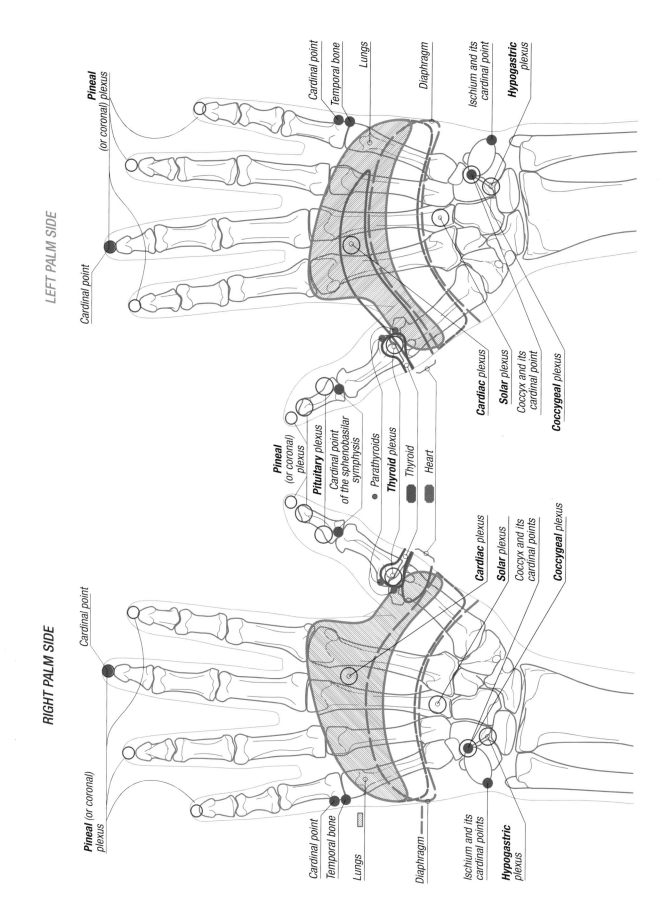

LEFT PALM SIDE

Pineal *(or coronal) plexus*

Cardinal point

Cardinal point

Temporal bone

Lungs

Diaphragm

Ischium and its cardinal point

Hypogastric *plexus*

Cardiac *plexus*

Solar *plexus*

Coccyx and its cardinal point

Coccygeal *plexus*

Pineal *(or coronal) plexus*

Pituitary *plexus*

Cardinal point of the sphenobasilar symphysis

• Parathyroids

Thyroid *plexus*

Thyroid

Heart

RIGHT PALM SIDE

Cardinal point

Pineal *(or coronal) plexus*

Cardinal point

Temporal bone

Lungs

Diaphragm

Ischium and its cardinal points

Hypogastric *plexus*

Cardiac *plexus*

Solar *plexus*

Coccyx and its cardinal points

Coccygeal *plexus*

Synthesis of the Plexuses, General Organs, and the Hormonal and Digestive Systems

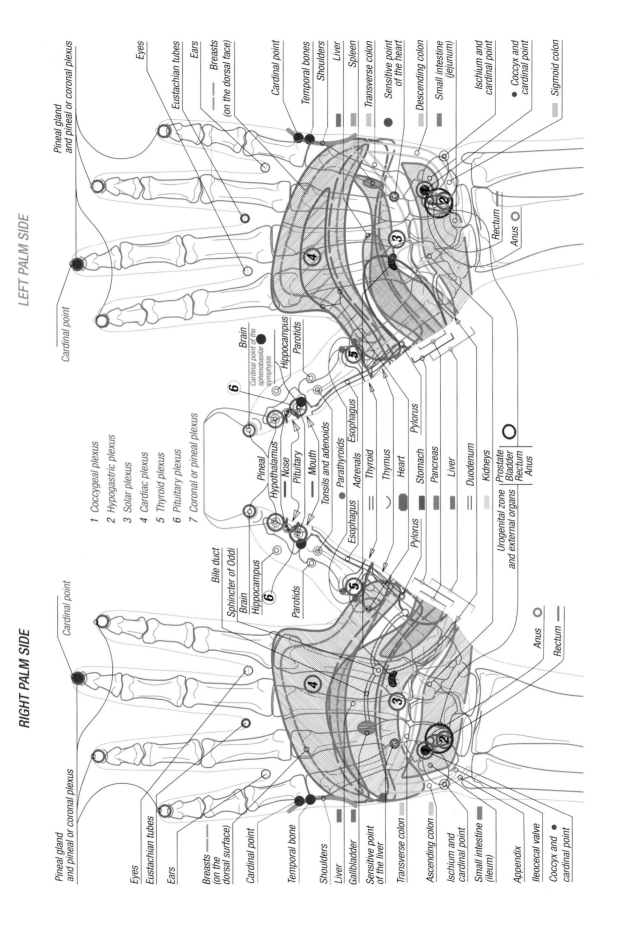

LEFT PALM SIDE

Pineal gland
and pineal or coronal plexus

Eyes

Eustachian tubes

Ears

Breasts
(on the dorsal face)

Cardinal point

Temporal bones

Shoulders

Liver

Spleen

Transverse colon

Sensitive point
of the heart

Descending colon

Small intestine
(jejunum)

Ischium and
cardinal point

Coccyx and
cardinal point

Sigmoid colon

Cardinal point

Rectum

Anus

1 Coccygeal plexus
2 Hypogastric plexus
3 Solar plexus
4 Cardiac plexus
5 Thyroid plexus
6 Pituitary plexus
7 Coronal or pineal plexus

Brain

Cardinal point of the
sphenobasilar
symphysis

Hippocampus

Parotids

Pineal

Hypothalamus

Nose

Pituitary

Mouth

Tonsils and adenoids

Esophagus

Parathyroids

Adrenals

Esophagus

Thyroid

Thymus

Pylorus

Heart

Stomach

Pancreas

Pylorus

Liver

Duodenum

Kidneys

Urogenital zone
and external organs

Prostate
Bladder
Rectum
Anus

Anus

Rectum

Bile duct

Sphincter of Oddi

Brain

Hippocampus

Parotids

RIGHT PALM SIDE

Cardinal point

Pineal gland
and pineal or coronal plexus

Eyes

Eustachian tubes

Ears

Breasts
(on the
dorsal surface)

Cardinal point

Temporal bone

Shoulders

Liver

Gallbladder

Sensitive point
of the liver

Transverse colon

Ascending colon

Ischium and
cardinal point

Small intestine
(ileum)

Appendix

Ileocecal valve

Coccyx and
cardinal point

The Solar Plexus: Digestion

This plexus can be found above the navel, and its reflex point on the hand—palm side up—is located in the inner edge of the third metacarpal. It is the seat of fear and anxiety. It governs digestion and corresponds to the pancreas and liver. It is the primary stabilizer of emotions and reactions.

Working on this plexus is helpful in the treatment of diabetes and hypoglycemia, general digestion, and the metabolizing of fats and sugar.

The Cardiac Plexus: Immune System

This plexus is located at the level of vertebra T4, and its reflex point can be found on the palm side of the hand, between the top of the second and third metacarpals. It forms the connection between the mind and the body. It is the first to be affected by stress and mental attitudes. This plexus is the protection center of the body and the immune system; it governs the circulation of lymph, growth, and muscle strength. It corresponds to the thymus.

Working on this plexus makes it possible to treat edema, muscles, and circulation, while stimulating the body's immune system defenses.

The Thyroid Plexus: Metabolism

This plexus is located in front of the trachea and its reflex point, looking at the palm of the hand, can be found at the base of the first phalanx of the thumb. It is connected to oral expression and controls calcium.

Treatment of this plexus is effective for all metabolic disorders, growth, spasmophilia (tendency toward convulsions or spasms), osteoporosis, arthritis, and osteoarthritis.

The Pituitary (or Hypophyseal) Plexus: Hormonal System

This plexus is located in the center of the forehead and its reflex point is on the middle of the second phalanx of the thumb, on the palm side of the hand. It controls body fluids such as blood and water, and it corresponds to the pituitary gland and the hypothalamus.

The purpose of treating this plexus is to restore balance to the entire hormonal system.

The Pineal or Coronal Plexus: Endocrine and Nervous Systems

This plexus is located in the center of the head at the third eye, and its reflex point is on the thumb (above the reflex points of the pituitary and hypothalamus). The pineal and related points can also be found on the pads of the other fingers. As the contact point between the endocrine system and the nervous system, the pineal gland distributes hormones to the hypothalamus and to the pituitary gland.

Working on this plexus helps treat both endocrine and nervous disorders. The application of deep pressure to these reflex points restores balance to plexus function, thereby helping to regulate the hormonal, immune, lymphatic and craniosacral systems. This in turn helps restore homeostasis to the entire body.

The Chakras and the Plexuses

The chakras, the subtle energy centers of the body, correspond to the plexuses, which are associated physiological centers. They too can be assessed to determine the state of a person's emotional and physical health. They can become damaged by a traumatic accident or emotional shock. The major chakras can be found in the middle of the palms of the hands as well as on the soles of the feet. See the location of the corresponding plexuses in the image on page 97 to determine where the chakras can be found on the hands.

The Chakras and the Plexuses

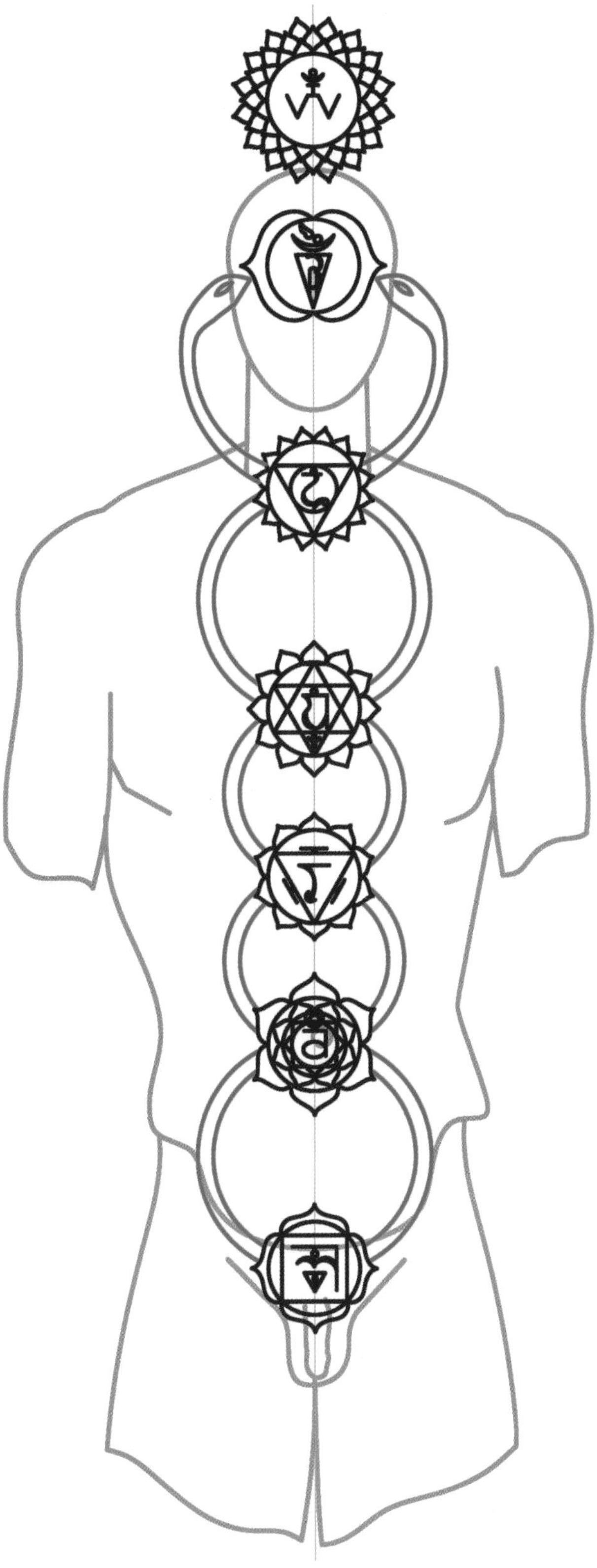

THE CHAKRAS

Sahasrara

Ajna

Vishuddha

Anahata

Manipura

Svadhisthana

Muladhara

THE PLEXUSES

Pineal or coronal

Pituitary

Thyroid

Cardiac

Solar

Hypogastric

Coccygeal

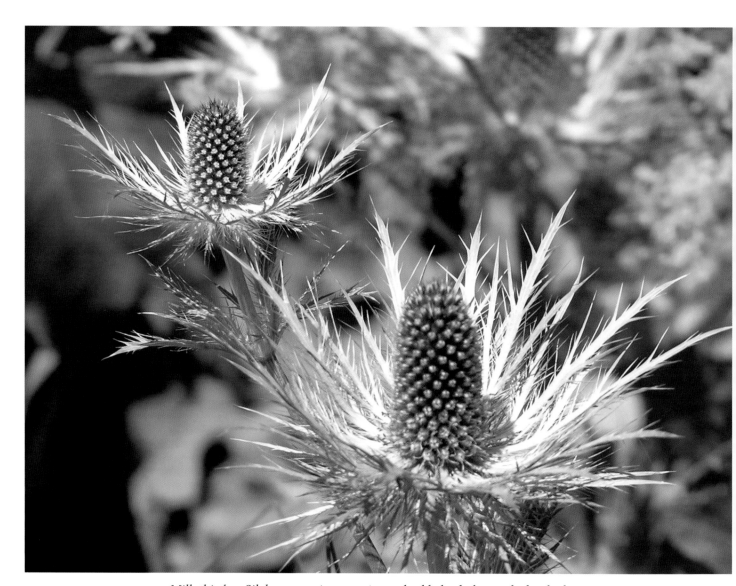

Milk thistle—Silybum marianum—is a valuable herbal remedy for the liver

PART FIVE

Beyond Reflexology

The Essence of Being

If the doors of perception were cleansed,
everything would appear to man as it is, infinite.

WILLIAM BLAKE,
THE MARRIAGE OF HEAVEN AND HELL

Live, but Live Well

Creating a Healthy Lifestyle

For some years now the average life span has been increasing. As a result, treating disease and degenerative conditions has increasingly become the common lot of therapists.

Aging begins in the brain. Studies of Alzheimer's disease have shown evidence of certain mechanisms that cause cerebral aging, that of memory in particular.

Water, the Essential Element

Water is the primary component of the human body. Water is the key element in respiration, perspiration, and the elimination of urine. Rainwater (without pollution), naturally gentle, is the best. Tap water is much harder and contains oxides. This is the reason why many people use filters to soften water and purify it of the nitrates that come from fertilizers, as well as chlorine and other toxic substances.

Drinking a cup of boiled water first thing in the morning encourages yang action, thereby inducing peristalsis. As a general rule, people drink warm or hot water when the body is cold. Ice cold water, on the other hand, can banish the effects of alcohol and lower body temperature in the case of fever; otherwise it is not advised. Room-temperature water is generally best to drink throughout the day for hydration.

Water Is the Best Medicine

Blood is primarily made up of water, red and white corpuscles in suspension, salts, proteins, and other components. Water is also present inside the cell. The protoplasm that surrounds the nucleus also contains a large quantity of fluid that ensures its proper functioning.

All forms of medicine are quite clear on the dangers posed by dehydration. Dry mouth, intense thirst, wrinkled skin, osteoporosis, osteoarthritis, and then, when dehydration becomes more serious, loss of consciousness and even death, are all signs and consequences of an imbalance in the hydric equilibrium of the body.

You need sufficient water to make saliva, which is 99.5 percent water. Normally, the body secretes two quarts of saliva a day. This saliva contains enzymes that are essential in beginning the process of digestion of dietary starches and fats. They also help break down food particles entrapped within dental crevices, protecting teeth from bacterial decay. In addition, saliva serves a lubricative function, wetting food and permitting the initiation of swallowing, and protecting the mucosal surfaces of the oral cavity from desiccation. The enzymes contained in saliva also reduce hemorrhaging and contribute to the synthesis of protein. As well, because it has antibacterial properties, saliva inhibits the growth of cancerous cells. Therefore, when saliva is insufficient in quantity—notably, as a result of dehydration—its functions are diminished.

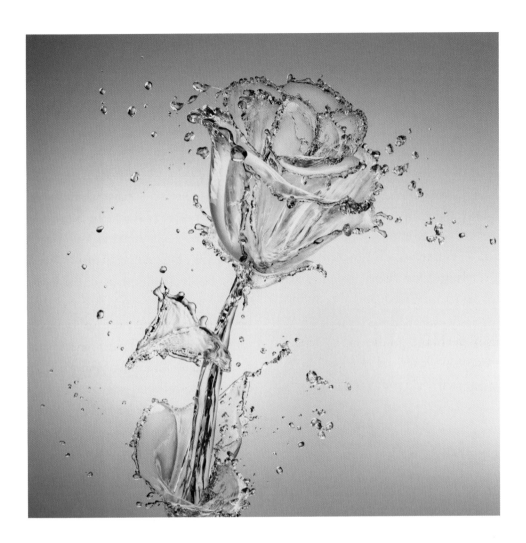

Eating Correctly

While an in-depth discussion of diet is beyond the scope of this book, the following are some general guidelines on eating correctly:

It is generally recommended that people eat a large breakfast, a moderate lunch, and a light dinner. Avoid overconsumption of alcohol, as well as stimulants, synthetic products, food substitutes, complicated preparations, sauces, and unhealthy food combinations. Eat small amounts of healthy food, chewing thoroughly, and strive to go four to five hours between meals. To stop hunger pangs, try drinking a glass of water between meals. Eat fruits before meals.

Problems like high cholesterol and high blood pressure, so prevalent today, must be examined in light of various factors, especially diet. It is certainly easier to measure cholesterol and blood pressure than to evaluate one's eating habits, and it is easier to prescribe medication rather than try to change someone's dietary habits. However, any strategy for preventing heart attack and its complications should, as a strict priority, begin by examining and adapting the dietary habits of people at risk. In fact, the more the relationship between cardiovascular disease and individual genetic factors is studied, the more we have come to realize that genetic factors are less important than lifestyle, especially diet. It has been found that so-called environmental factors—mainly, eating habits—are apparently the predominant culprit for those at risk.

The Power of Omega-3s

Forty-five years of clinical practice have led me to conclude that when there are large deficiencies to be addressed, food supplements are essential tools in restoring homeostasis to the organism. Food supplements can help address any number of acute and chronic conditions and all matters relating to general health including:

► fertility and puberty issues and menopause
► rheumatoid arthritis
► cardiovascular health
► asthma and allergies
► cancer
► mood disorders
► healthy brain and aging
► weight management

Fatty acids play a decisive role in one's health and are one of the first things to keep in mind these days because of the fact that our food has become so deficient in nutritional value. Understanding the power of omega-3s and fatty acids in general makes it easy to grasp their importance. My long years of experience and observation in a large number of clinical cases has often led me to prescribe vitamin E, lecithin, and omega-3 in the form of fish oil and evening primrose oil for a period of six months before disorders gradually vanish and homeostasis is restored.

Improvement of the daily diet is, of course, essential. Taking vitamin and mineral supplements should also be monitored, but the largest deficiencies involve fatty acids and their intestinal absorption. Reflexology and standard treatments of the digestive system contribute to their absorption and distribution, which has a direct effect on the brain and brain function, as well as on the immune, cardiovascular, and hormonal systems. Fats (lipids), including those supplied by foods, are important in medicine because they form the structure of our cellular membranes. The two primary lipid molecules are cholesterol and fatty acids.

Lipids and Cholesterol

Lipids are molecules that are averse to water, which is unable to dissolve them. To function, these molecules must therefore be organized in a particular way. This is why they are practically never "free" in our primary body fluids (the principal fluid being blood), but instead combine with other molecules or else organize themselves in more or less complex molecular structures until they form membranes. Lipids, along with proteins and carbohydrates, constitute the principal structural components of living cells, which also include fats, waxes, phospholipids, cerebrosides, and related and derived compounds.

Cholesterol has sparked an enormous amount of attention in contemporary medicine, whereas, oddly enough, fatty acids are relatively ignored despite the fact that they are, in mass and complexity, the most important lipids of living organisms. Cholesterol is a molecule that specifically appears in animals and is entirely absent in plants. Cholesterol is the precursor of numerous hormones involved in reproduction, therefore it is essential to the survival of species. It is essential for the absorption of dietary fats as it permits the formation of bile. For all these reasons, and also because it is easily measured in the bloodstream with the use of simple technology, dosing patients with cholesterol has been, along with the similar use of glucose, the first biological mixture used systematically in medicine to try to understand and prevent cardiovascular disease.

The discovery that a high level of cholesterol is statistically connected with the risk of cardiovascular disease and heart attack has prompted extensive studies on anticholesterol medications and foods. Yet fatty acids—both saturated and unsaturated—are of fundamental importance to both simple organisms (bacteria) or complex ones (mammals), as they provide the structure for all biological membranes, forming a "fluid mosaic" of which each square is a fatty acid. The popular argument in favor of reducing the quantity of saturated fats consumed has a partly erroneous medical and scientific basis that can be summed up in a single phrase: cholesterol theory. In fact, no study of nutritional intervention has ever been able to demonstrate that an anticholesterol diet based on the consumption of polyunsaturated plant fats has played any role whatsoever in the reduction of incidences of heart attack. In fact, it is well-known (although oftentimes hidden by the food and pharmaceutical industries) that some of these anticholesterol diets actually encourage the appearance of certain kinds of cancer.

Saturated vs. Unsaturated

Fatty acids, simple linear combinations of carbon atoms with an acid function at one end, are attached to molecules—cholesterol and glycerol—that neutralize the acid function. Fatty acids determine the properties of the cells. Some also serve as messengers (like hormones) between the tissues and the cells and help defend against attacks, most notably those of an infectious nature. Fatty acids are identified in accordance with their number of carbon atoms and the kind of bond between these atoms (simple or double), such as oleic acid in olive oil. Those that contain several double bonds are polyunsaturated, such as the linoleic acid (two double bonds) in sunflower and canola oil.

From Omega-3 to Omega-9

In addition to the omega-3s, there are also omega-6s, omega-7s, and omega-9s. The leader of the omega-9s is oleic acid, present in large quantity in olive and canola oils.

This fatty acid is highly resistant to oxygen, heat,

and ultraviolet rays, and thus reflects the physical properties of the olive tree and its resistance to climactic restrictions that allow it to endure.

FATTY ACIDS	PRIMARY FOOD SOURCES
Saturated	Animal products (butter, cream, meat, deli meats, cheese) Tropical oils (palm, palm-kernel, coconut, cocoa butter) Cookies, pastries
Monounsaturated	Olive, canola, peanut oils Hazelnuts, almonds, pistachios, avocado
Polyunsaturated: Omega-3s	canola, walnut, soy, flax, wheat germ oils some leafy green vegetables fatty fish (sardines, mackerel, tuna, salmon, etc.)
Polyunsaturated: Omega-6s	sunflower, corn, soy, walnut, sesame, grapeseed, safflower oils

Human cells are able to synthesize all the saturated fatty acids as well as oleic acid. Omega-7 acids are more characteristic of dairy products (as a result of rumination). Humans are incapable of synthesizing fatty acids with eighteen carbon atoms from the omega-3 and omega-6 series. These fatty acids are also known as essential fatty acids.

Why Are We Deficient in Omega-3s?

Essential fatty acids are crucial for the functioning of many living organisms and are indispensable for humans in maintaining a state of optimum health. They can be compared to vitamins, and as for those nutrients, there are a varying amounts of deficiencies, if not outright absences. When absorbed by the intestines, fatty acids can provide a source of energy for the muscles, they can be stored in the form of fat, or they can participate directly in the life of the cells by being incorporated into the membranes. Some organs have a particularly high quantity of fatty acids, independent of their energy aspects. This is the case, for example, for the brain or the thymus. More than 50 percent of brain mass consists of lipids, and more than 60 percent of these lipids are omega-3 fatty acids.

Just what does "essential" mean when we're talking about fatty acids? As our cells lack the means to introduce the double bonds on the level of carbons in omega–3 and omega–6 fatty acids, linoleic acid and alpha-linoleic acid cannot be obtained from any other fatty acid. Because they play a huge role in our health, they are therefore called "essential," and we should find a way to ingest them every day through our diet. Officially, there are only two essential fatty acids: linoleic acid (omega-6), and alpha-linoleic acid 5 ALA (omega-3). We are theoretically capable of synthesizing their more complex descendants such as the EPA and DHA acids of the omega-3 family, which are longer and have more double bonds and play a major role in health. However, in reality our ability to synthesize these substances is quite limited, especially during the later years of life. We depend on our food intake for the entire series of omega-3s, and not only for the first one in the series, alpha-linoleic acid. Therefore, our diet should include, in addition to alpha-linoleic acid, foods that are rich in fatty acids with very long chains. These are found almost exclusively in fatty fish (or in capsules of fish oil) and in the eggs of hens that have been fed flax seed, as well as in flaxseed (linseed), hemp seed, chia seeds, pumpkin seeds, sunflower seeds, certain leafy vegetables, and walnuts.

While essential fatty acids (linoleic and alpha-linoleic acid) must be ingested with our foods, they should be in balanced quantities, because in order to transform them into compounds with longer chains our cells must make use of the same biological pathways and enzymes; excessive intake of one will hinder the metabolism of the other. It is unanimously recognized that our contemporary diet is far too rich in linoleic acid omega-6 and much too poor in alpha-linoleic acid

omega-3. Therefore it is important to actively increase one's omega-3 intake.

A Source of Fuel and Energy

During any kind of extended fast we use up some of our fat reserves. Essential fatty acids are therefore not only essential for our daily activities (muscular effort, regulation of the body's internal temperature, etc.) but also constitute an important dietary reserve. But the real importance of fatty acids for our health stems from the fact that *they are the constituent elements of our cellular membranes*. These membranes isolate the cell from its surrounding environment and permit the cell to create functional units (mitochondria, nucleus) within it. The concentration of omega-3 fatty acids in the cellular membranes, especially the cardiac and cerebral membranes, determines the level at which these organs function and their degree of resistance to a number of stressful situations.

Based on the estimates produced by studies using radioactive markers, 75 percent of the alpha-linoleic acid absorbed by the body is burned by the muscles in order to produce energy, 15 to 20 percent is stored in the adipose tissues (creating energy reserves), and less than 5 percent is used by the cells. The activity of many cells varies based on the fatty-acid composition of their membranes. For example, blood platelets produce clots that prevent bleeding in the event of a vascular rupture. However, their degree of "reactivity" depends on the quantity of omega-3 fatty acids in their membranes. Another example concerns the electrical activity of the cardiac cells on which heart rhythm depends. This electrical activity will vary in accordance with the quantity of omega-3 fatty acids in the cardiac membranes. Moreover, certain psychiatric conditions, or one's general mood, greatly varies depending on the quantity of omega-3s present in the brain. Finally, neurons possess a better resistance to oxygen loss (for example, during a cerebral vascular event like a stroke) or other invasive attacks (mainly due to medications) when their membranes are enriched with omega-3.

Fighting Cardiovascular Diseases with Omega-3s

The great medical and scientific discovery of the end of last century lies in the demonstration of the existence of cardiovascular diseases, the scourge of the twentieth century (worse than the plague of the fourteenth century) as the result of the recent (and absurd) evolution of our lifestyle. And if there is any domain in medicine where we can be positively certain of the major role played by omega-3s, it is in the prevention of cardiovascular diseases.

Only two preemptive interventions, both nutritional in nature, have made it possible to reproduce ischemic preconditioning: the moderate consumption of alcohol and more importantly, the consumption of omega-3 fatty acids.

Omega-3s Inhibit Platelets

By their effect on the metabolizing of triglycerides, omega-3 fatty acids can also interfere with the paths of coagulation. We know that consumption of high levels of omega-3 will cause the duration of bleeding to lengthen much in the same way as the effects of aspirin. Consuming omega-3s is beneficial as it is necessary for the brain, but it should be taken in the right quantity and for the right amount of time. I recommend one to two tablets a day maximum (1100 mg fish oil or 700 mg straight omega-3s), with a one month break every six months.

Brain Structures and the Evolution of Consciousness

Materialist philosophy denies the existence of any nonphysical essence of the human being. Yet all cultural traditions, and even the experience of life itself, remind us that while it is obvious that we possess a physical body as well as thoughts and emotions, it is equally evident that we are also something else. The names given to this essential part of the human being are as diverse as the cultures that have described this aspect. We can use the term *self* here, as it is here where we feel we truly exist.

The time has come in these opening years of the twenty-first century to restore to our essence the full power it deserves. This shift is not merely philosophical, for if we can manage to realize our full potential, person by person, it will propel us toward a great revolution in human consciousness, one that will make it possible to naturally create an entirely new world, both for ourselves and for the whole of humanity.

During the course of our evolution human beings have progressively gone through different stages that represent an evolution of consciousness. It is in the ability to recognize these stages and the place we currently occupy in this evolution of consciousness that the possibility of real progress resides. By recognizing where we are in this process, we can achieve optimal growth as individuals and as a species and more effectively realize our indwelling potential for happiness, potency, creation, and freedom. For millennia, humanity, drawing from every life experience, has been moving forward on the path of an increasingly broader consciousness in a very organic way and through successive approximations. The less advanced one is, the larger the gaps as well as the greater the suffering; the more we evolve, the closer we come to the middle way, the path of well-being and bliss.

The human being must acquire greater emotional mastery by means of an enlightened mind. To achieve this goal it is first necessary to know from where we are starting. Just how well have we mastered our thoughts and emotions? The heart and the emotions have long been seen as being connected; the connection between the heart and the mind is less frequently recognized. It would seem that intelligence was reserved for the head. One then strives to mentally guide what takes place in our hearts, belly, and bodies—in short, in the confused and complex realm of feelings.

The Rational Mind

The mind is the headquarters of all thought processes. It is the seat of various complex processes that are a function of human intelligence.

- ▶ The mind transmits information received from outside.
- ▶ It understands directives in response to this transmitted information.
- ▶ It is capable of establishing mastery over one's entire life.

▶ It takes care of the physical body intelligently.

In previous centuries, the domain of the emotions was generally overlooked. One was supposed to not express them, to have them under complete control—by whatever means possible—if one wanted to be a "good" person. In fact, the collective consciousness of our species was not yet ready to examine the dynamics of the emotional body, and there was an obvious preference to act as if the emotions did not even exist, or at the very least, as if they were something "bad."

With the arrival of the major trend toward materialist thought at the beginning of the twentieth century it was generally believed that all activities of human intelligence took place in the head. And although studies of human intelligence have been performed in many scientific fields—medicine, biology, biochemistry, neurology, and so forth—the IQ test, originally developed in the early twentieth century, only measured the abilities of one part of the mind. The possibility of the existence of other parts of the mind was not considered, nor was the possibility that emotions interact with the mind. In general, science did not even consider that the emotions have a major influence on the quality of life to create a healthy, balanced person and a healthy society. It was generally considered a proven fact that the rational mind was strong enough to hold the emotions in check. The scientific world, up until relatively recent times, considered the emotions burdensome and disturbing, with no intrinsic value, and actually harmful to an "objective" scientific approach. In this model, the intellect was seen as the supreme authority.

So what happens to the emotions when denied in this way? The cycle of human emotions—unacknowledged, unexpressed, not communicated, and unmanaged—continues to unfold daily in the world in one form or another. Some people make decisions that are to their detriment; others suffer from an absence of creativity, while still others express their emotions in terms of a plethora of negative, destructive,

self-sabotaging, aggressive behavior and in the form of physical ailments and diseases. Thus the rational being we believe we are has surreptitiously transformed into a package of mismanaged and denied emotions. By awarding supremacy to the rational mind, the human being has been stripped of a very powerful source of energy: the emotions. In this way we have severed our connection to a potent source of innate intelligence and creativity.

Nevertheless, the dominant role that the rational intellect has held in the course of human evolution has not been a mistake. It comes from the effort that human consciousness made to transcend our primitive ancestors' earlier era of unrestrained emotionality. The emphasis on the rational has resulted in our modern culture, in which the intellectual aspect dominates. In more recent times, however, the human being has been put under the microscope again, this time to take our other aspects into account, namely, our emotions. Psychologists and social workers, grappling with the problems of their clients, were no longer able to ignore this emotional reality. In fact, the public at large requested this acknowledgment of our human emotions so that we can better handle the frustrations and stress that are an inherent part of our daily lives, especially with regard to relationships. Once the reality of the emotions and their impact is acknowledged, once we have learned to accept them rather than repress them, the challenge then becomes one of learning how to handle them most effectively. But what form of intelligence is best suited for managing the emotions to channel them in a positive way?

Emotional Intelligence

After glorifying the purely rational intelligence for quite some time, people of late have begun to recognize that the rational mind is no longer sufficient to allow us to grasp either the world of the human psyche or the material world. We are now talking about "emotional intelligence," also known as EQ—the emotional quotient. This refers to the ability of people to perceive and evaluate their own emotions and those of others, such that they can discriminate between different feelings and label them appropriately. In this way they can use emotional information to guide their thinking and behavior. The term was coined in 1995 by author, psychologist, and science journalist Daniel Goleman, who wrote a best-selling book by that title.

It is certain that this acknowledgment of the impact of the emotions represents a great leap forward, a significant opening in the prevailing system of materialist thought. It is an evolutionary leap from the paradigm ruled by the rational mind that has historically sought to deny this aspect of the human being. A growing number of organizations and businesses, both private and governmental, have become aware of the relational qualities of emotional intelligence and are acting on this newfound knowledge.

It is important to note that emotions are not intelligent in and of themselves. But they can be selected and used intelligently. They are an energy reservoir that when maintained in a pure, powerful, free, and well-managed state, can give people the possibility of living in a way that is wonderfully fair, balanced, creative, and loving. Just as recent discoveries in quantum physics have given an enormous boost to physical science and technology, the passage beyond rational and emotional intellects to other aspects of consciousness will make it possible to realize an extraordinary expansion of human potential.

The results of the many studies that have been conducted in the field of neurology have made it possible to precisely describe various physical circuits in the brain. It has been found that these circuits correspond to different types of conscious activities. Before going any further we should underscore the following scientifically proven fact, which is of utmost importance in this book: it is not the brain that generates consciousness, but quite the opposite; it is the level of the person's consciousness that determines what parts of the brain are activated. Furthermore, the body is extremely "true" and direct

in the ways it reacts. This is why the observation of its physical mechanisms is so useful for us in shedding light on certain phenomena of consciousness, and in facilitating a better understanding of our human nature.

The Limbic System, a Primitive Instinctive Circuit

For a very long time, primitive humans needed to possess a sure and rapid-fire way of reacting to ensure their survival. During this early era, a difference of several thousandths of a second in reaction time could be the difference between life and death. It so happens that to deal with these extreme situations and in the absence of a developed cerebral cortex, nature endowed humans with a primary shortcut that we all still carry inside us: the limbic system.

The limbic region is located inside the brain itself, in a region called the cerebral amygdala; it's like a brain within a brain. It possesses a specific way of dealing with information in accordance with three functions, for the essential purpose of guaranteeing survival. At the primitive level of evolution, these three mechanisms in the raw state had to work hard to fulfill their reason for being:

▶ fear (for maintaining safety)
▶ the reproductive instinct (for maintaining the continuation of the race)
▶ the protection of one's territory (for maintaining a survival space)

With these three mechanisms operating as guiding principles, all new information was treated in the following manner:

Information was recorded immediately and simultaneously on all levels in the primitive parts of the brain. This recording was precise and complete; it included all sensory perceptions, all the reactions of the physical body and consciousness (even if the

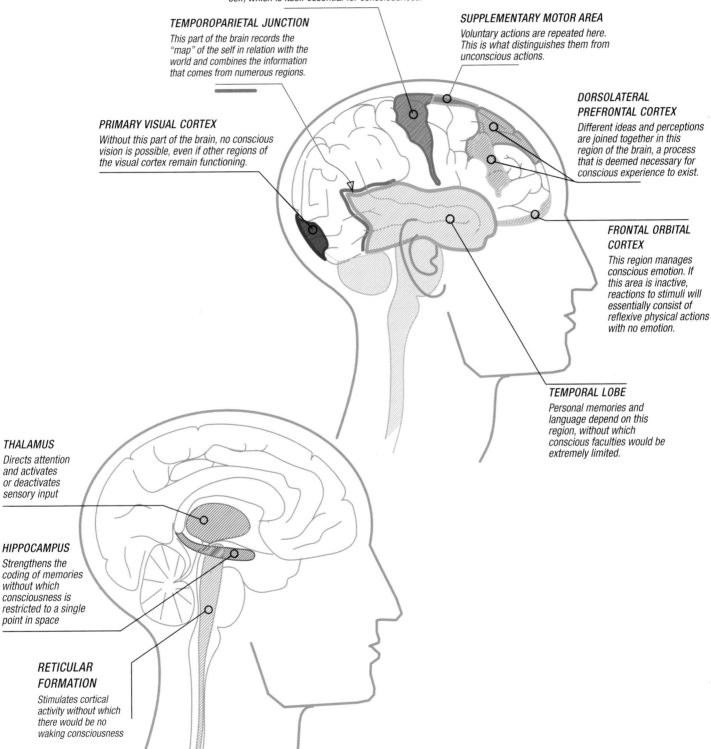

MOTOR CORTEX

Physical awareness (which involves the motor cortex) appears to be an essential element for the sense of self, which is itself essential for consciousness.

TEMPOROPARIETAL JUNCTION

This part of the brain records the "map" of the self in relation with the world and combines the information that comes from numerous regions.

SUPPLEMENTARY MOTOR AREA

Voluntary actions are repeated here. This is what distinguishes them from unconscious actions.

PRIMARY VISUAL CORTEX

Without this part of the brain, no conscious vision is possible, even if other regions of the visual cortex remain functioning.

DORSOLATERAL PREFRONTAL CORTEX

Different ideas and perceptions are joined together in this region of the brain, a process that is deemed necessary for conscious experience to exist.

FRONTAL ORBITAL CORTEX

This region manages conscious emotion. If this area is inactive, reactions to stimuli will essentially consist of reflexive physical actions with no emotion.

TEMPORAL LOBE

Personal memories and language depend on this region, without which conscious faculties would be extremely limited.

THALAMUS

Directs attention and activates or deactivates sensory input

HIPPOCAMPUS

Strengthens the coding of memories without which consciousness is restricted to a single point in space

RETICULAR FORMATION

Stimulates cortical activity without which there would be no waking consciousness

consciousness then was primitive), and of course all the controlled actions and gestures that guaranteed survival in the past. This is how the cerebral amygdala and the limbic system have become the keepers of a certain number of "memories" that are handed down from one generation to the next. For the moment, we can say that these memories come from a certain collective consciousness that is the bearer of the evolutionary process. They also come from more specific memories belonging the species' entire lineage, which every human being now carries. We learn through experience what assures our survival, and this information is recorded in this part of the brain. These memories are valuable, particularly those connected to the dangers that have been encountered and the reactions that permitted our ancestors to escape these dangers. They had to be, and remain, very easily accessible at any time, in a way that is quite rapid.

The mechanism of survival in action is therefore an action of recording, then assessing for similarities to previous experiences. It works this way: When a new situation manifests, the amygdala does not take time to analyze the situation in detail to obtain a clear, precise view of what is really happening. This is an emergency situation, and in order to overcome all eventualities and avoid all risks, the amygdala satisfies itself with crude, rapid perception of the situation so that it can determine if there is any similarity, even a vague one, between this situation and what is remembered of a previous situation. If in this rapid-fire way the amygdala determines that there is a similarity, however vague, it immediately orders the brain to make a series of automatic reactions identical to those that were used in past situations, as they had then guaranteed the person's survival. This recording-similarity mechanism is capable of activating the appropriate physical reactions in a split second. To a large extent these reactions can be compared to the instinctive reactions of animals. The reptilian brain is particularly involved in this case.

Conscious and Unconscious Emotions

Emotions are essentially unconscious physical reactions to the presence of danger or other circumstances. This is why, for example, the sight of a snake will automatically prompt the body to go on alert and flee. This response is ruled by the limbic system. As well, in human beings emotions are also consciously experienced as "feelings" that give meaning and value to life, however, these are reduced in the limbic system, which does not manage consciousness itself, only the fight-or-flight response.

The unconscious physiological component of emotion is generated in the deepest regions of the brain in the form of signals that are then transmitted to the body so that it can prepare itself to take action. In the case of consciously felt feelings, some signals activate the cortical regions, which has the effect of triggering the conscious feeling of an emotion. The type of emotion felt depends on the cortical regions that have been activated.

Moreover, the things that inspire an emotion attract our attention more quickly than other things that don't trigger an emotion. This is why we become aware of a threatening element much more quickly than a stimulus that does not trigger any emotion. This is connected to the fact that the amygdala unconsciously perceives the threat and alerts the conscious brain to be ready to receive an important perception. It should be noted that positive things also attract attention more rapidly than neutral things.

Desire and Reward

It is hard to define desire with any precision, but it may be described as the sometimes irrepressible wish to obtain something that will give us pleasure or satisfaction. There are circuits in the brain that are part of the limbic system that regulate desire and reward (i.e., the satisfaction of desire).

The desire to eat or to make love are survival values (all the various kinds of love have survival value), but these desires can be destructive if they become addictions. It seems that pleasure and desire follow different circuits, even though in both cases dopamine remains the principal neurotransmitter. It is released by the nucleus accumbens, the brain's "pleasure center" (which rules motivation, pleasure, and addiction), into the ventral tegmental area (VTA), a group of neurons located close to the midline on the floor of the midbrain and the source of dopaminergic cell bodies.

Strong sensations cannot fail to prompt a rise of adrenaline and dopamine in the cerebral circuits, hence the extreme activities like high-risk sports or dizzying amusement-park rides pursued by thrill seekers who wish to experience moments of intense pleasure. The feel-good hormone ocytocin, meanwhile, is produced by the hypothalamus and released by the stimulation of the sexual and reproductive organs during orgasm and childbirth. It triggers a sensation of well-being and encourages the formation of an attachment to the other person, in tandem with the release of vasopressin, with which it is closely connected. It also contributes to the treatment of social signs involved in the recognition of people and the construction of commonly shared memories.

The Intelligence Circuit

Over a period of thousands of years, right up to the present, humans have been developing another part of the brain, the cerebral cortex. Compared to the limbic system this is a more recent evolutionary development. This is the part of the brain that has been identified as the headquarters of mental intelligence, or at least a certain kind of intelligence. The development of the cortex coincides with an entirely new type of consciousness and a different way for humans to perceive reality. It is this cerebral cortex that is employed by modern humans and has permitted the installation of the ego, among other things.

In the intelligence circuit, information that is recorded by the senses, after traveling through the limbic brain, is transferred into the cerebral cortex, whose function is to take control of the situation in accordance with its own perception criteria. The human being is expected to become "rational" and "objective." The more instinctive areas of the brain should only be used to assist the intelligent cortex. The reactions induced this way should be all the more pertinent, as the cortex is believed to perceive reality more clearly. This is nonetheless a relatively slow route, slower than that of the brain's limbic areas. In fact, in this more developed region of the brain, information is analyzed and dealt with by a very large number of nerve circuits, which are responsible for the cortex's refinement but also account for the fact that it processes things more slowly than the first circuit, the amygdala. I emphasize this relative slowness of the neocortex in comparison to that of the limbic brain because this fact is significant once we examine another form of consciousness, a "third brain" that offers resources that are quicker and more reliable than those that this part of our intelligence can provide.

The Mental-Emotional Hybrid Circuit

The fact that the cerebral cortex evolved over a long period of time does not mean that it has brought about a reduction or elimination of the functioning of the amygdala or limbic regions of the brain. The dynamic of recording dangerous situations that the person survived thanks to an immediate and appropriate fight-or-flight response, which proved extremely useful during an earlier evolutionary phase, was not brought to a halt just because a thinking brain began to emerge. The amygdala continued to function as a lookout for all things pertaining to physical survival, and as the cortex emerged it further adapted and expanded its functions to embrace the new situations that arose as our emotional and mental bodies developed and along with that, the ego.

In this evolution, the amygdala retained its primary

role as a "protector," essentially against all forms of suffering, as human beings do not enjoy suffering. However thanks to the emergence of the ego it has expanded its recording system to memorize not only stressful situations engendered by physical threats but also all events that cause psychological stress, which is to say mental or emotional suffering. We suffer because we feel judged, rejected, forsaken, abused, or a victim of injustice. We suffer when we fail, when we do not obtain what we want, when we experience heartbreak or feel alone, powerless, or guilty—all kinds of experiences that our cavemen ancestors did not have to concern themselves with. In fact, the psychological survival mechanism is identical to the primitive mechanism for physical survival. This means that the two primary operating principles of the limbic system, recording-similarity, are extended and applied to all the situations a modern psychological human being may encounter in daily life.

On the recording side, every time there is stress or emotional suffering, the memory is imprinted (with the strength of the imprint proportional to the intensity of the stress) in order to guarantee the best possible outcome with regard to protecting the ego, along with the physical, emotional, and mental aspects of the being. Next, the principle of similarity is applied. The amygdala is completely averse to risk and is satisfied with an utterly vague similarity to unleash a succession of reactions, feelings, thoughts, and, ultimately, actions, all based on the source memory. Thus from the moment of the recording, the amygdala, like a powerful computer, continuously examines every current situation in order to compare it to a physical or psychological situation that occurred in the past. If the cortex, although more highly evolved, is not yet strong or developed enough, or if the memory contacted is too charged, then the amygdala and limbic system take control, causing physical, emotional, and mental reactions based on memories and not on an accurate and clear perception of the reality of the present moment.

This means that our hybrid emotional-mental response circuit is fairly automatic, vague, imprecise, and disproportionate, and thus much like the physical reaction of a primitive human. But this reality generally goes unrealized by most of us. Thus we have the same emotional, irrational reactions as in the past, the same ways of thinking and perceiving things (equally irrationally), the same reactions in our bodies as before, and in this way we repeat the past. Were the earlier reactions irritating, painful, unpleasant? It doesn't matter; what is important is to react as was done in the past and to use the psychological defense system that was then implemented, because we survived—or so we think.

It is this kind of reaction that still characterizes human beings most of the time at the current level of consciousness—and most of us are completely unaware of it.

But What Is the Cortex Doing At Times Like These?

In fact, the recording of memories takes place in two forms in modern humans. We are in the presence of a "double brain," each with its own way of dealing with information.

The cortex records facts as they are without any emotional charge. This happens, for example, during the acquisition of knowledge or, more generally, during neutral or pleasant experiences, those involving no stress or suffering, simply by observing, learning, and relaxed experiencing, therefore at times when energy is circulating freely. This is the seat of our memories that hold no emotional charge, those known as "free memories." This is also the brain that makes self-awareness possible.

The limbic brain is the headquarters of active memories. It is in this area of the brain that not only the event but the emotional charge connected to it are recorded. I call this "active" because these kinds of experiences are always ready to be "activated" by the most minor triggering element. Knowing their specific origin, whether it is personal (in the present or from a

CINGULATE CORTEX

This is area of the brain closest to the limbic system. It performs difficult tasks; deep-set desires or violent anger increases the activity of the anterior cingulate cortex. This region also comes into play when a mother hears her child crying. It contains a particular kind of neuron: the fusiform cells that play a dominant role in the perception of other peoples' feelings and the way one reacts to their emotions.

HYPOTHALAMUS AND MAMMILLARY BODIES

The hypothalamus is a tiny cerebral structure whose activity is both extensive and complex. An emitter and receiver of hormones, it has an influence on the body's reactions to its environment and is the source of emotions. It can also come into play in the fear reaction prompted by the amygdala. The mammillary bodies connected to the hippocampus by the fornix sit at the junction of memory and emotions.

FRONTAL CORTEX

The information arriving from the limbic system is transmitted to the frontal cortex to produce conscious feelings, whereas the conscious feelings about the environment are sent from the cortex to the limbic system, which thereby forms a cycle. The effects of an emotion on a thought are therefore stronger than the effects of thought on an emotion.

CORPUS CALLOSUM

The corpus callosum plays an essential role in the transmission of emotions between the two hemispheres. Women have a higher quantity of fibers in the corpus callosum than men. This explains the difference between the sexes in the realm of emotional response.

STRIA TERMINALIS

This part of the cerebral network connects the amygdala to other regions of the brain. It comes into play in responses to anxiety and stress. Cellular density differs in accordance with sex; it has thereby been shown that among transsexuals the cellular structure corresponds to the characteristic patterns of the sex into which they have chosen to change.

OLFACTORY TRACT

The olfactory bulb directs odorous messages directly into the limbic regions, whereas the signals of the other senses travel through the thalamus before coming back into the cortex. This is why odors inspire an intense emotional response instantaneously. The olfactory tract is the original emotional center and probably developed before the visual and auditory cortex.

THALAMUS

The thalamus, the center that selects among all information that enters the brain, is more or less involved in all activities. However, some thalamus nodes have a very powerful influence on the emotions because they transmit their important emotional stimuli on toward the appropriate limbic regions, such as the amygdala or olfactory tract, so they can be dealt with and change.

AMYGDALA

The amygdala is a tiny cerebral structure involved in emotions. It analyzes the degree of threat and the emotional meaning of internal and external information.

HIPPOCAMPUS

The hippocampus primarily comes into play with matters pertaining to coding and the resurgence of memories. Personal memories (episodic) display an emotional component. By recalling these memories, the hippocampus causes the reemergence of past emotions that can blend with present emotions or take the upper hand. This is how a sad memory can cast a pall over a moment of joy.

past life), ancestral, or from the collective unconscious is not essential. It is necessary, though, to acknowledge their existence in order to confront them appropriately.

There are two facts worth noting here:

How fast the information is dealt with: The very substance of these two kinds of brains is different. The physical matter of the neocortex is made from highly organized layers of neurons that allow for a slower but more sophisticated analysis of data. That of the limbic brain is formed more from a jumble of neurons based on a more primitive structure, which permits only one perception of reality. On the other hand, the limbic brain does allow for much quicker circulation of information and response time. We do know in fact that the limbic brain is capable of dealing with 40 billion bits of information a second, whereas the consciousness circuit that travels through the normal cortex can only deal with 2,000 bits a second. We need something that will let us catch up to this speed if we want to live without being at the mercy of unconscious charges. And it just so happens that something of this nature exists.

The power of creation: The slowness of the cortex is compensated by the fact that it has the ability to create in a free and original fashion, whereas the programmed and automatic amygdala can only reproduce the past and transmit information. Thus the cortex, although with its own limits, opens a completely different path that with the help of higher evolutionary developments will provide access to another way of perceiving reality, thereby offering humans greater freedom.

We still have a long road to travel and many major discoveries to make. According to neuroscience researchers, the current average human being is conscious of only 5 percent of his or her daily activities, and the other 95 percent comes from the person's unconscious program—and these figures are considered rather optimistic.

This is how these active memories generate not only emotional reactions but also different ways of thinking. This is why we can speak of an automatic mind that functions like a computer preprogrammed by the past. It needs to be readily understood that it is the emotional charge that permitted its recording in the person's mental region, and thus became automatic instead of intelligent. We think we are intelligent because several areas of our cortex enjoy more sophisticated development, reason in particular. But we are far from attaining mastery over it, even when dealing with the simple ups and downs of everyday life.

We therefore own a supercomputer within, constructed from emotional-mental material whose activity, unduly expanded, disproportionately applies the primary limbic-system mechanism of recording-similarity. This computer, whose full justification for existing occurred during the onset of human evolution when the cortex was in a very embryonic state, is now holding human beings in an illusory, restricted, ineffective world that is the source of much unpleasantness, if not great suffering. Where is emotional intelligence to be found? Certainly not here. This explains why the average human consciousness, despite the development of the cortex, still operates most of the time in accordance with the primary survival principles of our cave-dwelling ancestors. And this extends into psychological functioning; the recordings are a bit more complex and sophisticated, but the basic mechanism remains the same. On this level of functioning, the ego—in its still automatic form—is king.

Thus the three primary survival mechanisms—fear, the reproductive instinct, and territoriality—have adapted to our current psychological world and have led to three very specific forms of behavior: fear, pleasure, and power. As Annie Marquier, founder of the Institute for Personal Growth and author of *The Heart Revolution, The Power of Free-Will,* and *Free Your True Self,* explains, this is why, despite the development of human intelligence over thousands of years of evolution, this

List of Disrupted Functions

FRONTAL LOBE

Loss of simple movement of certain
    parts of the body
Inability to organize certain complex
    movements
Loss of fluidity in relation to other
    connected movements
Loss of mental flexibility
Persistence of single-mindedness
Mood changes
Change of social behavior or
    personality
Difficulty in problem-solving
Inability to make correct oral
    expressions

TEMPORAL LOBE

Difficulty in recognizing known objects
Difficulty understanding some spoken
    words
Difficulty choosing between things
    seen or heard
Difficulty in identifying and verbally
    expressing certain objects
Loss of immediate memory
Interference with long-term memory
Increase or decrease of sexual drive
Inability to catalog common objects
Logorrhea (incoherent talkativeness
    due to right lobe deterioration)
Increase of aggressive pride

BRAIN STEM

Difficulty swallowing
Difficulty in perception and
    organization of perception of the
    environment
Disequilibrium problems in movement
Nausea and vertigo
Sleeping difficulties
Sleep apnea

PARIETAL LOBE

Inability to concentrate on several
    objects at the same time
Inability to remember the name of an
    object
Forget words when writing
Difficulty reading
Difficulty drawing
Difficulty telling right from left
Difficulty performing mathematical
    exercises
Absence of sensation or its localization
    in certain parts of the body
Inability to focus on a given point
Difficulty in hand-eye coordination

OCCIPITAL LOBE

Visual disruption
Difficulty placing objects
Difficulty identifying colors
Hallucinations
Visual illusions and inability to see
    certain objects
Inability to see some written words
Difficulty recognizing certain objects
    either present or drawn

CEREBELLUM

Loss or inability of coordinating delicate
    movements
Inability to walk
Inability to reach certain objects
Trembling
Dizzy spells
Difficulty in the coordination of
    language
Inability to make rapid movements

intelligence still remains for the vast majority of human beings in the service of our more basic drives. What is worse is the fact that this intelligence can make the destructive effects of these primitive mechanisms even more formidable.

Consciousness and Freedom

We can take the first steps toward higher consciousness and freedom. First, we must begin to become conscious of the self, of our thoughts and emotions. This is not always pleasant, in fact far from it! Yet it is on this level that we can begin to consciously experience the battle between the cortex-ruled intelligence and the primitive emotional-mind body. We all certainly want to hold on to the joy and pleasure we feel when our desires are satisfied, but what are we to do with fear, sorrow, anger, and other so-called negative emotions? As a general rule, these negative emotions are repressed. Only the cortex is strong enough to inhibit the amygdala. However, we know that the amygdala does not make this easy for the cortex, and repressed emotions can pop back up to the surface just when they are least expected. Here I am referring to the feelings that come from the limbic brain that can be quite strong, which direct the majority of people in the world today.

Repressed, unacknowledged emotions usually have health consequences. For example, fatigue, which a large number of people experience today, is often due to the fact that the unconscious, which is charged with repressed and suppressed emotional material, uses all the energy it can get to perform its tasks twenty-four hours a day. The majority of cases of work exhaustion today actually stem from this conflict between the rational mind, which has its own desires, ambitions, and social, relational, and familial needs, and the limbic brain, which, burdened with its own fears and desires, resists and strives to ensure that things take place in accordance with its memories and not otherwise.

It is often the case that the most petty choices of daily life as well as the major decisions made during the course of a lifetime are determined not by the intelligent and loving will of our true essential being, but by a survival mechanism programmed in the past. When this happens, freedom is lost because this mechanism makes the person a slave to the emotions.

Fear, the first primary mechanism of the limbic system, is essentially a state of separation—from one's true self, from others, and from Spirit or Source. Most people today are in a state of insecurity and stress generated by fear. The second primary mechanism of this primitive system, desire, manifests as greed and a craving for pleasure that generates a permanent state of dissatisfaction and a predatory attitude. The egotistical quest for power, the third primary mechanism, generates combativeness, competition, domination, violence, jealousy, fanaticism, and hatred. Any of these mechanisms generate a state of separation. To get out of this cycle of negative emotions you have to recognize their source. Every time you tell yourself: "It is stronger than me," it is because a memory from the automatic mind has been reactivated. There are ways to get out of this painful cycle; recognizing the source is the first step. The need for psychological nourishment has been added to the need for physical nourishment.

Contrary to what one might think, the automatic mechanisms of the limbic system do not just function occasionally. It is not necessary to be in a state of stress, experiencing an emotional crisis, or in a state of panic, for the memories held in the amygdala to gain the upper hand. The limbic system functions twenty-four hours a day. This means that the average human being who has no self-awareness is constantly under its influence. In fact, we could even say that the more developed the mind, the greater the risk for the daily consequences of these emotional mechanisms to be harmful, as they are camouflaged, protected, and nurtured all the more skillfully by the power of the mind, thereby reinforcing the false individuality of the programmed ego.

The experience of the present moment is inaccessible as long as we remain in the lower circuit of consciousness. On the other hand, the blissful experience of the present moment is immediately available when we function out of a completely different circuit, out of another level of consciousness.

Love through Union

The search for love is in fact an intense quest for finding the lost sense of unity or oneness. Insofar as the intent of the ego left to its own devices is to reify a sense of separation in order to ensure the survival of the individual organism, love is certainly not part of its program. A direct and concrete expression of unity, love cannot exist in the reality of the lower circuit. This is not because the ego is evil; it is because it is a machine and true happiness is not part of its program. Therefore, our suffering stops in proportion to our increased ability to utilize another circuit of consciousness, that in which love exists.

Even if this automatic structure we carry inside is a source of many limitations, it is far from being useless. If we understand how to use it to our advantage, it can help us create extraordinary things. So we will hold on to our computer-brain. On the other hand, we shall no longer allow it to go beyond its duties. We will update it on a regular basis, consciously adding new memories to it that consist of the things we learned intentionally and the development of our talents. The evolution of the cortex—what we call *ego*—particularly in its mental aspect, is a positive event in our evolution. The intellect is a unique privilege of being human. It is in fact this intellect that can open the path toward something grand; it can be the bridge between the personality, the ego, and the deep self, the fully realized human being. The continuing evolution of human consciousness lies in humans' ability to create, and this creative aspect is a function of the intellect. Thus it is through the intellect, transformed and realigned, that we can truly experience the ecstasy of life in the union of hope and matter.

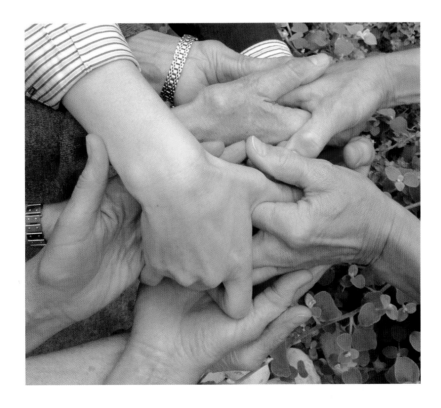

The Importance of Working with the Vital Force

Every living being possesses an intelligent vital force that preserves and maintains the cohesion (which is as spiritual and psychic as it is material) of his or her constituent cells. This vital life force is life, an attribute of the spirit, the inner physician, intuition, common sense, and so forth. Humans are the beings that make the least use of this force, thereby twisting the laws of life.

Kirlian photography, a collection of photographic techniques used to capture the phenomenon of electrical coronal discharges, makes it possible to see a person's electromagnetic field, or aura. In this way we can see all the changes caused by mental and emotional states. In this way too we can see changes in the electromagnetic fields of the cells in cases of psychosomatic disease, as this is an expression of the vital force. Here it is important to note that illness is a necessary stage on the path to healing. Its action can appear destructive, whereas it is actually constructive in that what is involved is a rebalancing of the energy in the person.

Under the effect of a strong emotion, a shock, stress, or a disease organism like a virus, the vital force is the first thing to be disrupted. This triggers an electromagnetic change that stimulates the body's defense mechanism, puts the autonomic nervous system in play, and causes a series of physical, emotional, and/or mental reactions. In short, in the same way that the electromagnetic field penetrates matter, the vital force penetrates an organism on every level.

Therapies that use the vital force such as acupuncture, homeopathy, phytotherapy, and reflexology act directly—slowly but completely, depending on the degree of tissue permeability—to restore the vital force. The tissues of the organism are the instruments, but only the vital force can heal. It is this force that determines what the body's priorities are based on the needs of the person.

The immune defense mechanism is affected by four factors:

▶ hereditary influences
▶ infectious diseases
▶ immune-depressant treatments and vaccinations
▶ the poor condition of the biological terrain (malnutrition, stress, etc.)

Any of these conditions can bring about a deterioration of all the body's systems.

In alternative and natural therapies it is recognized that different forms of energy—for example, a disease organism or a homeopathic medicine—can alter the patient's vital force, either negatively or positively depending on the type of energy. But just what is this force that dwells inside people and keeps them alive?

Polarity Theory

Polarity therapy recognizes the importance of the flow and balance of energy in the body, and its techniques involve balancing this flow to improve or maintain health. Developed in the late nineteenth century by Randolph Stone, a chiropractor and osteopath, polarity therapy is also known as *polarity balancing* and *polarity energy balancing*.

Polarity therapy theory suggests that there are four dimensions of human energy, which mirror the cardinal directions of the Earth: North, South, East, West. These should all function without any blockages, which are caused by stress, disease, or traumatic events. Bodywork to balance energy flow and restore health to the body is the most significant aspect of polarity therapy. The therapist views the body as a magnet with a positive charge on top and a negative charge at the bottom. Likewise, the therapist's hands have a positive electrical charge in the right hand and a negative charge in the left one. When placed on specific places, the hands can have a stimulating

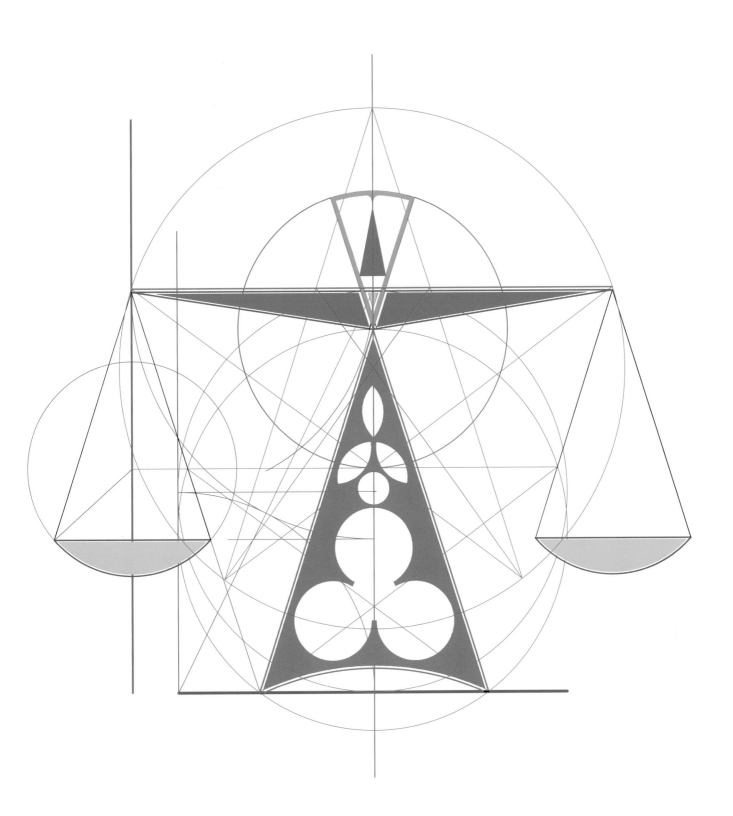

or calming effect. They stimulate the circulation of energy and balance the corporeal energy field.

We can look at tissues, cells, molecules, and atoms as elementary electromagnetic particles of the body that together communicate in a secret language whose meaning we are just beginning to understand. The aura, or biological electromagnetic field, could be understood as being the sum total of all an organism's energies. This part of the body is in direct and constant contact with the others. Could all this chemical, mechanical, electrical, and electromagnetic communication be energy? This is at least the basis of the principle of holistic unity, or homeostasis, which is the aim of reflexology.

From Reflex to Consciousness

Health, both yours and your patients', is a complex matter requiring attention, care, and reflection. Waking up to a happy thought, feeling the joy of being alive no matter what the circumstances are, is a state of mind that will result in the establishment of primordial balance, which equals health. Harmony of thought (creative spirit), sleep (regular rhythm of days and nights), and a balanced diet are all things that need to be maintained, retained, or acquired in order to enjoy good health.

Some people are born optimistic, happy to be alive, cheerful, loving, enthusiastic, and full of life; they are indeed lucky. Others take a more pessimistic view of things, and this causes them to form different mental habits that lead to their creating another kind of reality. In such cases, reflexology is a formidable tool that can help remedy this state of affairs as naturally as possible.

Homeostasis comes from the Greek words *homoios,* meaning "similar," and *stasis,* "position," which together designate balance and harmony between the body, mind, and emotions. The imbalance of just one component can cause a disruption of the others if this harmony is missing, given the fact that all the systems are interdependent. The objective of reflexology is to restore this balance, which is often disrupted by environmental, physical, psychological, or social agents. In this way, we possess an invaluable tool for promoting a complete state of physical, mental, and emotional well-being.

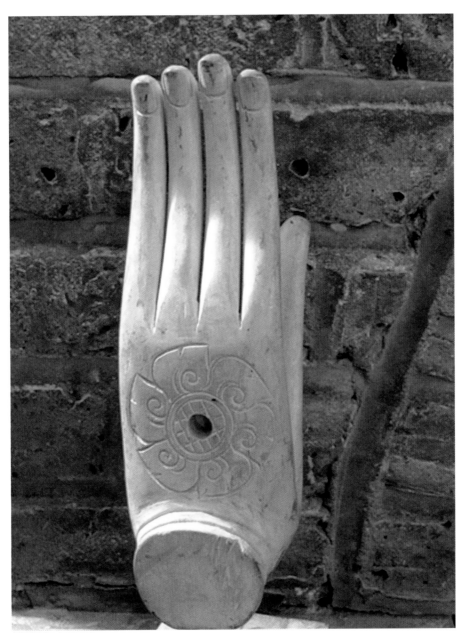

Wooden sculpture from Indonesia—posterior face of the hand

About the Author

During the course of her medical studies in London, which included earning a degree in osteopathy, Dr. Martine Faure-Alderson realized that above and beyond the basic premises of all the various medical disciplines is the idea that the human being is an interconnected whole. This led her to pursue more extensive studies of various natural therapies, including naturopathy, acupuncture, phytotherapy, and homeopathy, for the next twenty-five years, both in England and in South America.

Doreen Bayly, the author of *Reflexology Today* (Healing Arts Press, 1984), first introduced Dr. Faure-Alderson to reflexology in the 1960s. Bayly had been a student of Eunice Ingham (1889–1974), a pioneering physiotherapist who published extensively on the subject of zone therapy as a result of her extensive research in the 1930s. At this time when she encountered the science of reflexology, Dr. Faure-Alderson was working in a clinic where several of her patients were suffering from digestive disorders. She decided to work on the zones of the feet that correspond with digestion as part of her treatment of these patients. Three months of testing were sufficient to demonstrate the effectiveness of reflexology. This led to her decision to conduct specific clinical studies with Doreen Bayly.

In 1968, Dr. Faure-Alderson began teaching reflexology in a seminar setting. Her medical training enabled her to provide a scientific perspective on the efficacy of reflexology, which until that time had only been supported by anecdotal evidence. It also allowed her to provide the necessary level of precision in determining the exact placement of the points on the feet and hands that correspond with this or that organ or area of the body, which in turn allowed her to provide a more precise diagnosis and "reflex treatment" of the disorders afflicting her patients.

The global nature of the view she strove to apply in her diagnoses and treatments of various conditions—a view that encompasses the nature of the person's consciousness as well as its physical, psychological, and mental antecedents—inspired her to found her Paris-based school, the Faure-Alderson Total Reflexology Therapy School (RTTFA, i.e., Réflexologie Thérapie Totale Faure-Alderson), in 1974.

Throughout the 1970s, Dr. Faure-Alderson undertook the task of integrating into her practice the ideas of Hans Selye (1907–1982), a pioneering Austrian-Canadian endocrinologist who conducted much important scientific work on the stress response. She also confirmed the importance of occipital zones in foot reflexes. Armed with the results gained through her practice, she discovered the zones on the hands and the feet that correspond with those of the brain. During the 1990s she pursued a course of research with her students that allowed her to top off her distinctive method with the understanding of the role that craniosacral therapy could play in foot reflexology. She integrated key elements of this discipline into her own practice, with a particular focus on the effect of the primary respiratory mechanism (PRM) and cerebrospinal fluid on the cranial nerves and the three levels of being (mental, emotional, and physical).

Gradually, thanks to the insights gained through her extensive practice, studies, and teaching, she was able to incorporate other branches of alternative medicine, including naturopathy, homeopathy, and acupuncture, into her standard treatment protocol. She thereby created a synthesis of all the natural therapies, giving her RTTFA method a solid multidisciplinary foundation. It is this multidisciplinary approach that makes the reflexology method of Dr. Faure-Alderson a truly global therapy.

Today Dr. Faure-Alderson teaches and lectures worldwide, in the United States, Canada, Australia, New Zealand, and Europe.

Total Reflexology Training Seminars

The Cranio-Sacral Reflexology International training is a two-year course. The first year is devoted to a complete, meticulous study of anatomy, physiology, and illness. Time is also made available for the practice of reflexology. The second year is devoted to the full training of the student in reflexology, including the protocols for the craniosacral, lymphatic, immune, cardiovascular, and autonomic nervous systems. A certificate is awarded upon completion attesting to the quality of the student's work.

This training course is complemented by an annual series of postgraduate lectures for the purpose of honing the skills of reflexologists. The studies include the natural medicines, puberty and menopause, the three levels of being, the emotional being in reflexology, the facial bones and reflexology in the domain of ear, nose, and throat medicine, and hand reflexology.

Contacts

Paris, France
Danielle Vidy-RTTFA, secretary, treasurer—administration
Administrative address:
11, rue du Haut Soleil
52150, Soulaucourt-sur-Mouzon
Telephone: +33 3 25 31 13 85
E-mail: rttfaoffice@gmail.com
Website: ww.w.ecole.faure.alderson.fr

London, England
CSRI Academy of Excellence
Administrative Address:
187 Ember Lane,
East Molesey
KT8 0BU

Canada
Académie de Réflexologie Crânio-Sacrée (Quebec), Quebec Branch of the RTTFA
Administrative address:
Barbara Smithwick
1652, rue Royale
Trois Rivières, QC
G9A 4K3
Telephone: 819-375-0939

Administrative address:
Ildiko Zambo
100 Blvd. Harwood
Bureau 001
Vaudreuil-Dorion, QC
J7V 1X9
Telephone: 450-219-1911 or 514-883-9836

Or to find craniaosacral reflexology, brain, and other courses near you,
e-mail
admin@craniosacralreflexologyinternational.com
or visit
www. craniosacralreflexologyinternational.com

Bibliography

Atlas d'anatomie humaine: La Grand Larouuse du cerveau [Atlas of Human Anatomy: The Grand Larousse of the Brain]. Paris: Larousse, 2010.

Bayly, Doreen E. *Reflexology Today: The Stimulation of the Body's Healing Forces through Foot Massage.* Rochester, Vt.: Healing Arts Press, 1984.

Brouillet, Dennis, and Arielle Syssau. *La maladie d'Alzheimer: Mémoire et vieillissement* [Alzheimer's Disease: Memory and Aging]. Paris: Presses Universitaires de France, 2000.

Carter, Rita. *Mapping the Mind,* rev. ed. Berkeley, Calif.: University of California Press, 2010.

Chopra, Deepak. *Life After Death: The Burden of Proof.* New York: Random House, 2008.

Davidson, John. *The Web of Life.* Saffron Walden, UK: C. W. Daniel Co., 1988.

De Mello, Anthony. *Awareness: The Perils and Opportunities of Reality.* New York: Doubleday, 1992.

Faure-Alderson, Martine. *Total Reflexology: The Reflex Points for Physical, Emotional, and Psychological Healing.* Rochester, Vt.: Healing Arts Press, 2008.

Guo, Bisong, and Andrew Powell. *Listen to Your Body: The Wisdom of Dao.* Honolulu, Hawaii.: University of Hawai'i Press, 2001.

Israël, Lucien. *Cerveau droit cerveau gauche: Cultures et civilizations* [Right Brain, Left Brain: Cultures and Civilizations]. Paris: Plon, 1995.

Issartel, Lionel, and Martine Issartel. *L'Ostéopathie exactement* [Osteopathy, on the Dot]. Paris: Robert Laffont, 1983.

Janet, Jacques. *La Médecine Biodynamique* [Biodynamic Medicine]. Paris: Editions R. Jollois, 1999.

Kunz, Barbara and Kevin. *Manuel complet de réflexologie pour les mains et pour les pieds* [Complete Manual of Reflexology for the Hands and the Feet]. Paris: Ed. France Loisirs, 2004.

Labonté, Marie Lise, and Guy Corneau. *Se Guérir autrement, c'est possible, comment j'ai vaincu ma maladie* [Other Ways of Healing Are Possible: How I Conquered My Illness]. Montreal: Editions de l'Homme, 2001.

Magoun, Harold Ives. *Ostéopathie dans le champ cranien* [Osteopathy in the Cranial Field]. Paris: Sully, 2000.

Marquier, Anne. *Le maître dans le coeur* [The Teacher in the Heart]. Montreal: Editions Valinor, 2007.

Piveteau, Jean. *Le main et l'hominisation* [The Hand and Anthropogenesis]. Paris: Masson, 1991.

Schuenke, E., E. Schulte, and U. Schumacher. *THIEME Atlas of Anatomy: Head and Neuroanatomy.* Stuttgart, New York: Georg Thieme Verlag, 2007.

Seignalet, Jean, and Henri Joyeux. *L'alimentation, ou la troisième médecine* [Diet, or the Third Medicine]. Monaco: Rocher, 2012.

Servan-Schreiber, David. *The Instinct to Heal: Curing Depression, Anxiety and Stress without Drugs and without Talk Therapy,* repr. ed. Emmaus, Pa.: Rodale, 2005.

Thieffry, Stéphane. *La main de l'homme* [The Human Hand]. Paris: Hachette, 1973.

Upledger, John. *A Brain Is Born: Exploring the Birth and Development of the Central Nervous System.* Berkeley, Calif.: North Atlantic Books, 1996.

———. *Your Inner Physician and You: Craniosacral Therapy and Somatoemotional Release.* Berkeley, Calif.: North Atlantic Books, 1997.

Upledger, John, and Vredevoogd. *Craniosacral Therapy.* Seattle, Wa.: Eastland Press, 1983.

Véret, Patrick, and Parquer, Yvonne. *Traité de Nutripuncture* [Treatise on Nutripuncture]. Méolans-Revel, France: Désiris, 2005.

Walker, Kristine. *Hand Reflexology: A Textbook for Students.* 2nd ed. London: Quay Books, 2000.

List of Plates

Index

Page numbers in *italics* indicate illustrations.

Books of Related Interest

Total Reflexology
The Reflex Points for Physical, Emotional, and Psychological Healing
by Martine Faure-Alderson, D.O.

The Reflexology Manual
An Easy-to-Use Illustrated Guide to the Healing Zones of the Hands and Feet
by Pauline Wills

Trigger Point Therapy for Myofascial Pain
The Practice of Informed Touch
by Donna Finando, L.Ac., L.M.T., and Steven Finando, Ph.D., L.Ac.

Trigger Point Self-Care Manual
For Pain-Free Movement
by Donna Finando, L.Ac., L.M.T.

The Encyclopedia of Healing Points
The Home Guide to Acupoint Treatment
by Roger Dalet, M.D.

The Reflexology Atlas
by Bernard C. Kolster, M.D. and Astrid Waskowiak, M.D.

Facial Reflexology
A Self-Care Manual
by Marie-France Muller, M.D., N.D., Ph.D.

Gemstone Reflexology
by Nora Kircher

INNER TRADITIONS • BEAR & COMPANY
P.O. Box 388
Rochester, VT 05767
1-800-246-8648
www.InnerTraditions.com

Or contact your local bookseller